MASTER MENOPAUSE WITH GRACE

CONQUER SYMPTOMS OF HOT FLASHES, WEIGHT GAIN, POOR SLEEP AND MORE; NAVIGATE EMOTIONAL UPS & DOWNS, AND REKINDLE INTIMACY WITHOUT FEELING OVERWHELMED

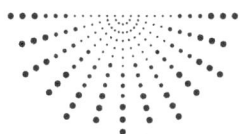

MAYA BLOOM

© **Copyright 2024 - All rights reserved.**

The content contained within this book may not be reproduced, duplicated or transmitted without direct written permission from the author or the publisher.

Under no circumstances will any blame or legal responsibility be held against the publisher, or author, for any damages, reparation, or monetary loss due to the information contained within this book. Either directly or indirectly. You are responsible for your own choices, actions, and results.

Legal Notice:

This book is copyright protected. This book is only for personal use. You cannot amend, distribute, sell, use, quote or paraphrase any part, or the content within this book, without the consent of the author or publisher.

Disclaimer Notice:

Please note the information contained within this document is for educational and entertainment purposes only. All effort has been executed to present accurate, up to date, and reliable, complete information. No warranties of any kind are declared or implied. Readers acknowledge that the author is not engaging in the rendering of legal, financial, medical or professional advice. The content within this book has been derived from various sources. Please consult a licensed professional before attempting any techniques outlined in this book.

By reading this document, the reader agrees that under no circumstances is the author responsible for any losses, direct or indirect, which are incurred as a result of the use of the information contained within this document, including, but not limited to, — errors, omissions, or inaccuracies.

CONTENTS

Introduction	v
1. THE MENOPAUSE METAMORPHOSIS - WHAT REALLY HAPPENS?	1
The Science Simplified	3
Timeline of Transition	13
Global Glimpse	16
2. SYMPTOM SPECTRUM - FROM MILD TO WILD	22
The Big 7: Usual Suspects of Menopause	23
The Undercover Agents of Menopause	31
Severity and Span of symptoms	38
3. NAVIGATE THE EMOTIONAL ROLLERCOASTER	41
Map the Emotional Terrain	42
Depression and Menopause	46
Anxiety's Grip	48
Empowerment through Self-Care	49
Build Resilience and Emotional Muscle	55
4. SAILING SMOOTH - RELATIONSHIPS & MENOPAUSE	61
Intimate Insights	62
Family and Friends	67
Social Circles and Workplaces	71
5. NATURE'S NURTURING - HOLISTIC HEALING	76
What is Holistic Healing?	76
Herbal Heroes: Nature's Healing Wonders	80
Mindful Methods	83
Therapeutic Touch	86
Understand HRT: Explore its Risks and Benefits	90

6. NOURISH AND FLOURISH THROUGH
   MENOPAUSE   95
   Metabolism shift: Understand the slowdown   96
   Power Foods: Boost Hormonal Harmony and
   Energy   97
   Foods to Forsake   100

7. LIFE AFTER MENOPAUSE - THE PROMISED
   LAND   114
   When do you know you've made it?   115
   Does life go back to normal after menopause?   119
   Let's get to the good part!   120

   Conclusion   125
   Notes   129
   Bibliography   131

INTRODUCTION

Becoming

> *Natural, universal, and transient*
> *Among all women born,*
> *Yet treated like the plague,*
> *Avoided, perhaps worse,*
> *For the symptoms are not sores or boils,*
> *But a subtle shift, at first, and then...*
> *Fierce,*
> *Like the full moon of life's passage,*
> *Immense power,*
> *Making oceans leap and wolves howl,*
> *The semi-final cycle,*
> *Preparing the bearer for the next phase,*
> *Bestowing the feathered cap of eternal wisdom.*

∼

In my 20s and 30s, and even in my early 40s, I frequently dismissed menopause as something that would happen to other people. Since I have always been a fit and healthy woman - who has thankfully never really suffered from any significant ailments - I felt that somehow mother nature would give me a free pass. I would skip that part of life's journey and somehow live eternally in the body I was, that the 'big change' was not meant for me.

Then it happened: the hot flashes, the night sweats, the sudden (and I do mean sudden) weight gain, and, of course, the hormonal roller coaster that we have all been warned about. It reminded me of going through puberty - that physiological change that you cannot escape, no matter how badly you resist it.

Coping with mood swings, anxiety, and irritability became a daily reality, and insomnia suddenly plagued me - the girl who could once sleep 8 or even 10 or 12 hours, without a problem. My memory started letting me down; "perhaps this is a good thing," I thought. Maybe it will help me forget the way that I almost bit my partner's head off after he innocently reached out for a cuddle in the middle of one of my internal 'moments' - I practically slapped his hand away! Nothing felt the same; my closest people started feeling like strangers.

After suffering in silence (apart from the occasional outburst when I couldn't control my tongue or the deluge of tears that would appear out of nowhere when I least wanted to deal with it), for what felt like an eternity, I started speaking to a few of my friends. I wasn't coping; I was worried; what was happening to me? Something had to give, or else…

Fast forward about seven years, and I look back, wishing I was just a little bit more prepared for the journey of menopause. Once I understood what was happening, I could start looking for effective strategies to alleviate the physical discomfort and emotional distress. I was almost relieved when I found out that I was going through menopause. At least I wasn't perishing from some mysterious condition that was turning me into a version of myself that I did not want to be or get to know.

I've often heard that 'knowledge is power,' and I began to understand this when I finally regained a sense of control over my body and my emotions. Learning techniques to once again achieve restful sleep was a complete game changer; my overall well-being increased, and I could feel the vitality return to my being. Regaining focus and cognitive sharpness was a relief; for a moment there, I was worried that there was something seriously wrong with my brain; my husband even (half-jokingly) suggested that I see a neurologist after I had forgotten full-blown conversations that we had had for the umpteenth time.

More than knowledge, through the many, many conversations I had with friends, sisters, mothers, grandmothers, and any random woman who would indulge me in a chat about their personal experience with menopause, I started feeling like I was part of a community: a tribe of women who were going through this together. We could share experiences, advice, wisdom, and most of all, as I learned by watching women who had completed their journey, we could look forward to a great treasure at the end of the menopause rainbow…

That is my story, and because of how profoundly the process impacted me, I started thinking about sharing what I have learned, hoping that it will help other women navigate their menopause journey a little bit better. I sincerely believe that the more we normalize speaking about this transformational period in every woman's life, the more we will be able to unlock the incredible support network that should, in my view, be available to every woman going through menopause. Here's the thing: the safer we feel sharing our stories and talking about our experiences, the more we feel comfortable exploring the subject, and the more we can tap into the deep well of wisdom that is the collective knowledge of an army of post-menopausal women.

That is why, in the pages ahead, you will find a journey of understanding, embracing, and thriving (yes, thriving!) during your time of transformation - of going through the change. If you are anything like me, and you find yourself caught off guard by the unexpected intensity of the experience, this book will guide you through the process of coming to terms with yet another aspect of the natural metamorphosis of womanhood.

Menopause is completely natural, and I believe that we urgently need to shift our perspective and create a change in how the world sees menopause and menopausal women. You have probably come across a news article or two about a woman who was dismissed from her employment because she was not performing well enough because she was dealing with menopause, and most of us have been in situations where women are made fun of because of their symptoms. Personally, I've seen it too many times and it irks me every time. How is it okay that women are ridiculed and mistreated just because we are going through this natural change? I believe it is time to turn things around and it really is up to us to bring about a change in how menopause is treated, and this book is my contribution to this change.

How will this book help you? The first step is to understand what menopause is, to really grasp the scientific intricacies of hormonal shifts from perimenopause to postmenopause and to begin to understand why menopause is an integral part of a woman's life and what the evolutionary advantages of this profound transition is.

Once you understand where the symptoms of menopause come from and what other women are going through, it becomes much easier to manage, and it also helps us feel less isolated. That is why, in the pages of this book, you will find real stories of women who have been where you are now; you will also find insights, advice, and practical solutions that have been tried and tested.

Before we can start a revolution, we need to feel good in our bodies and have the mental, emotional, and physical strength to stand up for ourselves and our right to age gracefully.

Here's the thing: menopause isn't just a physical transition; it carries profound emotional and psychological dimensions, and again, we need to learn how to navigate this, we need to stop blaming ourselves for having unpleasant emotions, otherwise we will remain at war with ourselves and the world around us. We have to learn to love ourselves through this, and then we can also learn to remain loving to our partners, family, friends, and colleagues so that we can maintain healthy relationships.

How do you love yourself when the way you are feeling and sometimes behaving seems so unlovable? I believe that the only way to do this is to take a holistic approach, looking at the whole being and the individual circumstances of every woman, and then crafting a lifestyle plan to support the person through their journey. Luckily today, even Western women are increasingly drawn to holistic approaches for managing menopause and no longer just relying on Hormone Replacement Therapy (HRT); we are working on healing our hormones that have been hijacked by our modern lifestyles, food, and even medicine.

Speaking of food, I have learned that the food we eat is so closely linked to the state of our hormone health. In the West, medical doctors are seldom *au fait* with the latest information on diet, and we simply have to do our own research in this regard and every woman will benefit from crafting an optimal diet that supports her through this journey. I've done much of that research for you and I have even prepared a diet specifically to help manage hormonal shifts.

At the end of the menopause-tunnel, there is a bright light, the potential for a new beginning in your life - a new stage of self-knowledge which you can navigate towards from day one - and a future which has the potential to be better than you ever imagined.

I look forward to sharing this journey with you, and together, we'll embrace the wisdom, resilience, and strength that this portion of your life will bring you. Let us normalize conversations about this profound period in every woman's life, and tap into the deep knowledge and experience shared by all of us.

Thank you for joining me. My wish is that this book will empower you through this journey and leave you feeling graceful, beautiful, vibrant and lovable, always.

Maya Bloom

1
THE MENOPAUSE METAMORPHOSIS - WHAT REALLY HAPPENS?

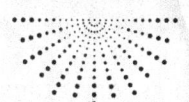

The circle nearly complete now,
Marking the third birth of the feminine,
First she is born, the transition from otherworld to this
The first breath, establishing connection to earth,
Cutting of the cord, disconnected from the womb,
and into a world of contrast, the human experience.
Next follows the transition from child to woman,
A rite of passage some say, turmoil,
And uncomfortable process, growing into a new being
Now she, too, can bring life to earth.
And enjoy a season of fertile birthing of new creation.
Then comes the time for the third transition;
From mother to Sage,
A season of wisdom enters.
A new creature emerges,
A becoming, not a birthing.
Becoming the essence of who you are,
You smile softly,
You have walked through the fires of your own hell,

And created paradise.

◈

*I*n this chapter, it is my mission to help you start seeing menopause as a natural change. We will look at the scientific intricacies of hormonal shifts all the way from perimenopause to postmenopause. I will also talk about why menopause is an integral part of a woman's life and why it should be seen as an evolutionary advantage.

Here's the thing: like the first paragraph of the poem in the introduction says, menopause is natural and transient, and it is also universal. This means, if you are a woman, this is a phase you will inevitably go through... there's no doubt about that, it is not something that you can sidestep. I do believe, though, after my personal experiences and those of so many other women, that it is empowering knowing that when you equip yourself with information - take the insights I have shared in this book for instance - the process can become much more manageable.

I will do my utmost to demystify menopause for you. When I used to think about menopause, I thought of an abstract picture of an old woman, hunched over, covered in cloth, hiding her face and body as much as she could. Today, thankfully, this picture has changed completely. I now see menopause for what it is: a natural metamorphosis brought on by hormonal shifts, moving the woman through the stages from perimenopause to postmenopause.

"Metamorphosis," you may ask, what metamorphosis? If you are like a younger version of me, you may assume that there is no real life after menopause. You are not alone. My heart breaks every time I think of a conversation that I had with a close friend. She is a strong, fierce woman, and while we are close friends, I have always joked that I am a little bit afraid of her; she questions everything and says it as it is. This is a woman that defies excuses and gets things done. On that particular day however, she looked me in the eyes, and she said to me that she was sure she no longer had a purpose in this world. She said, 'Now that my eggs have dried up, I am useless to the world.'

Hearing this initially made me worried that I would become 'useless' or insignificant once I went through menopause; I was terrified of this idea, and while the words seemed very real coming from my friend, she had had a harrowing experience, I knew that could not be the truth. Why would the creator design us women in such a flawed way? Are we truly designed to become like the walking dead on this planet when we are, at one point, the most powerful of creators, the only ones of our species that can bring new life into this world?

I decided that I would not rest until I figured out how it all fits together and why we were made to go through the change known as menopause. What I found is that right there at the end of that rainbow is the real pot of gold, a version of you that you could not imagine from your current vantage point, an experience of life so rich, that when you find yourself in it, you will know that the process of change was not only a necessary evolution but a gift that you would never return. We will uncover the layers of this gift as we move along; I can't give it all away right here in Chapter 1.

What follows is an explanation of the process of menopause, starting with the hormonal changes that bring on menopause.

THE SCIENCE SIMPLIFIED

Hormonal Overhaul

In the words of one of my friends (she is the funny one): "I don't know what's going on with my body. It's like my hormones have decided to throw a party, and no one told me, the host of the party."

"Hormonal Havoc" is what menopause is synonymous with. Hormones are chemical messengers that tell your body how to function during menopause and during the period leading up to it, as well as after it; several hormonal changes occur in our bodies as we go through the menopausal change. The three main Menopause hormones are Estrogen, Progesterone, and Testosterone. Of course, the hormonal effects are not the only physiological changes that will occur; and there are other hormonal influences beyond these. Still, they are the key characters on the proverbial dancefloor of 'the Menopause dance.'

Estrogen's Ebb and Flow

Let's start with the lead dancer in the hormonal disco party, estrogen. After the onset of menopause, levels of estrogen slowly diminish to equilibrate with those of age-matched men.

What is Estrogen? Estrogens are a group of hormones, and they play an essential role in your regular sexual and reproductive development; they are also known as 'sex hormones.'

Estrogen's main job is to regulate your menstrual cycle, and it also affects your reproductive and urinary tract, your heart and blood vessels, your bones, breasts, skin, hair, mucous membranes, pelvic muscles, and even your brain.

While your ovaries produce most estrogen hormones, your adrenal glands and fat cells also create small amounts of estrogen in your reproductive years.

Then, what happens as you get older?

Firstly, it is important to understand that estrogen levels will rise and fall throughout your life; this is entirely normal. As you get older, your estrogen levels diminish, and eventually, your ovaries will stop producing estrogen, and your menstrual cycle stops. While your ovaries have stopped producing estrogen, your fat cells will now produce estrogen instead, but it is a different kind of estrogen. The primary form of estrogen in your body now switches from estradiol (produced primarily in your ovaries) to estrone (produced primarily in body fat), and this switch, together with lower estrogen levels overall, can lead to, among others, painful sex, lower sexual desire, and hot flashes.

Progesterone's Role

Just as every dancer needs a partner, estrogen has its counterpart, namely progesterone. Progesterone supports menstruation, and it also helps your body maintain a pregnancy, specifically in the early stages.

The primary function of progesterone is to prepare the lining of your uterus for a fertilized egg to implant. If you do not fall pregnant, the endometrium sheds in the form of your menstrual period. If a pregnancy does occur, progesterone waltzes in like a knight in shining armor to support the pregnancy.

A gland called the corpus luteum is mainly responsible for producing progesterone. This is a temporary gland, and it only develops after your egg is released from your ovaries (ovulation). It is responsible for maintaining progesterone levels after conception and fertilization. Your adrenal glands and placenta also make progesterone.

During pregnancy, progesterone levels will get higher and higher in each trimester, up to its climax in the third trimester, when you are in weeks 28 to 40 of your pregnancy. When ovulation stops, the knight knows he is no longer needed; he takes a bow, and leaves the arena. Your progesterone levels decrease in the years leading up to menopause, when ovulation stops.

Testosterone's Subtle Shifts

When you think of female hormones you normally do not pay much attention to the role of testosterone, right? That is because we have been taught that testosterone is a 'Man's Hormone' and there are many cultural and political opinions that make us shy away from embracing testosterone as an essential part of our make-up. The fact is that testosterone is one of a woman's primary sex hormones! How's that? When I first heard about this, I was utterly confused, so I had to do more research.

Although people know it primarily as a male sex hormone, females also need certain levels of testosterone. In females, most testosterone converts into the sex hormone estradiol.

Let's look at testosterone in both men and women, to get a better understanding of its working.

We start by looking where testosterone is produced. In men, it is mainly the testes that produce testosterone, and in women it is mainly the ovaries. In both sexes, the adrenal glands are also responsible for producing small amounts of testosterone.

So, in men, testosterone is important for: Development during puberty, creating sperm, strengthening bones and muscles, brain development and functioning, keeping their hearts healthy, and keeping their sex drive high.

In women testosterone is the hormone that adds that subtle groove to the party, holding the baseline of the music and it is essential for maintaining the levels of other hormones, our sex drive and fertility. It's also essential in making new blood cells, for our brain health, heart health and, like men, strengthening muscles and bones. For both men and women, there is a strong link between low sex drive and fertility and low testosterone.

Here's some more information about testosterone in women that may help you understand it better: Let's start with a fact that few of us know: Women produce three times as much testosterone as estrogen before menopause. Let that sink in! Such a radical shift is sure to have a massive effect on our overall functioning.

Let's look at testosterone more closely: Our bodies naturally transform testosterone into oestradiol, a primary growth hormone for female reproductive organs and normal breast development and the changes your body goes through in puberty. It also maintains the eggs in our ovaries and is responsible for ovulation. In addition, it helps you maintain bone health, it has neuroprotective properties, and it improves blood flow through your body.

So, what can we expect to happen to our bodies when our testosterone takes a plunge? In terms of physical symptoms, as our levels of testosterone gradually decline during the menopause process, we may experience lower libido, one of the most worrying menopause symptoms for many of us, and in Chapter 4, we will have a closer look at how to deal with this. Here are some of the other symptoms that you may experience as testosterone levels in your body drops: low energy and tiredness, decrease in muscle tone and strength, lowered fertility, irregular menstrual cycle, vaginal dryness, mood changes such as feeling depressed or anxious, and even thinning hair.

I know that this sounds daunting, but rest assured that this book is designed to help you thrive through these changes. It is possible to go through menopause gracefully and emerge as a better version of yourself, and you take the first step by understanding what your body is doing.

Ovulation's End

One of the most significant moments in the menopausal dance is the end of ovulation. It's like the DJ finally turning off the music at the party.

The connection between the end of ovulation and finally reaching a state of menopause lies in the gradual decline of ovarian function as women age. Let's have a look at how it works: When you are born, your ovaries have around one million immature eggs called primordial follicles. Throughout your life, the number of eggs decreases, and by the time you reach menopause, less than 1000 eggs are left. As we age, our ovaries produce fewer and fewer viable eggs, ovulation becomes less frequent, and our menstrual cycles become irregular. Eventually, our ovaries stop releasing eggs altogether, and ovulation stops completely. At this point, we are longer able to conceive.

Case Study - When menopause comes knocking

In this case study, I want to introduce you to two of my closest friends. Let's call one of them Anna and the other Marylin. Both of them are around the same age, and they both started their menopause around the age of 40. Both of them are from a middle-class background, as we would call it, and both have jobs and family responsibilities.

Anna is an avid runner, having completed many marathons in her life, and Marylin is a dancer and has stayed fit throughout her life by spending time in the ballet studio.

Both women had vibrant health before menopause and had active, energetic lifestyles, but ended up having very different menopause experiences:

When Anna was around 40, she started losing sleep and experienced sudden hot flashes. She also started gaining weight, despite her regular running routine. She was perplexed because she didn't understand what was happening, she didn't change her diet or lifestyle but her body was responding differently than it had before.

Marylin, at the same time also started feeling out of sorts. She had always been finely attuned to her body, and when she started noticing unexpected heat in her body and a shift in her body composition, she started questioning what was going on and soon realized that it was probably the onset of menopause.

Anna, being a 'get on with it' type of person, who does not spend much time on self-care but instead pushes through obstacles, was so busy with life that she tried to ignore these early symptoms and became really hard on herself for not being able to control her weight and moods like she used to. She would openly chastise herself for being 'fat and lazy', and went into war with her body when it no longer responded the way she expected it to.

Marylin, conversely, knew from the research she had done, that the symptoms were not going to simply disappear, and that she had to take charge of what was going on in her body. As a first step, she went to her GP and shared her symptoms and concerns with her. The doctor ordered some simple tests to see if it was indeed menopause and she did a few extra tests to check if there were any serious underlying conditions. Once the test results came back, Marylin could relax, she knew that there was nothing wrong with her, and that it was merely time for her to flow into her menopause journey. She relaxed and started working on a menopause mastery plan with a mission to turn menopause into her personal muse, although at first she did not even know what this would mean.

Anna, on the other hand, just carried on with life as usual. She didn't see her doctor until a couple of years later when she became truly desperate. She tried working out more, and she took medicine to treat individual symptoms, all in an effort to get through each day as best she could while inside she was spinning out of control and her life felt like it was falling apart. She often asked herself why she couldn't just hold it together like she used to, feeling like a failure every time she did this.

In Anna's personal life, there was havoc, she was in constant battle with her husband, the mood swings and loss of libido caused friction between them, and the kids became anxious feeling the constant tension between their parents. At work, things were difficult. She was a high-powered attorney, but now she could barely contain her feelings, and she would cry at the most inappropriate times and shout at staff when small things went wrong. She no longer recognized herself.

In Marylin's world, while the same changes occurred, she had a very different life experience. She started carefully looking at treatment options and lifestyle changes that would help her sail through the changes smoothly. Some worked well, and some not so well, while yet others (like hormone therapy) were not options she wanted to consider unless as a last resort. She already had a morning and evening routine of self-care, gentle movement, focused breathing, and meditation, and she fine-tuned that to help her stay connected to her body through the changes.

Marylin also sat down with her partner to explain the changes to him, and she explained to him how he would be affected and how things in their relationship and intimate life might change. Her husband became a partner in her menopause journey and would often come home with a small gift like a handheld water fan to help with her hot flashes or a tub of blueberries because he read somewhere that it may help with one of her symptoms.

Both these women, as you can see, went through more or less the same symptoms when their menopause started, but the way in which they approached it meant that they ended up having very different experiences. This comparative case study of my two dear friends is what motivated me to slow down and take charge of my own journey, so that I would thrive, instead of floundering in the face of menopause.

Biological Body Clock - timing of menopause

Menopause isn't a one-time event; it unfolds gradually, akin to a beautifully choreographed performance.

As you approach menopause, in other words, the end of your menstruation, or more accurately, the point or date at which it has been 12 months after your last menstrual period (the official start of menopause), the changing hormonal levels in your body will give you telltale signs of what is happening in your body. Symptoms like hot flashes and night sweats, cold flashes, vaginal dryness, and discomfort during sex, which we will look at more closely in Chapter 2.

The process leading up to menopause varies for each woman; for many women, premenopause, also called perimenopause, will start around the age of 40 or even a bit before that, while menopause typically occurs around age 50, with the usual range being between 46-54 years. This being said, some women only reach menopause in their sixties, and as we will see below, some can go through menopause as early as their thirties.

Premature Menopause: Causes and Consequences

When menopause comes knocking before you turn 40, you go through something called "premature menopause". When it happens between the ages of 40 and 45, it is called "early menopause". In the west, around 5% of women experience early menopause, and about 1% experience premature menopause.

External Influencers: Factors accelerating menopause

So, why do some people go through menopause earlier than others, and can you control that at all? Here's what I found: Just as an unexpected gust of wind can speed up a dance, various factors in your life can either bring on the early arrival of menopausal changes or delay it a bit. Here's a summary of the most prevalent causes of the early or premature onset of menopause:

Family History: According to a study of 10,606 women, 37.5% of women who experienced early menopause had a family history of menopause before age forty-six years in either a mother, sister, aunt, or grandmother, compared to only 9% in the control group. If you have a sister who's had an earlier menopause, that is one of the strongest indicators that you may have the same experience. [1]

Smoking: If you are currently smoking, your risk for early menopause is double that of someone who has never smoked. The more you smoke, the higher this risk is, but the great news is that even if you were a heavy smoker before, your risk will decrease after you stop smoking. If you smoked lightly in the past, you are unlikely to have a higher risk for early menopause, according to a 2018 study.

[2]**Chemotherapy or Radiation:** Cancer treatments, like chemotherapy or radiation, can cause early menopause because they are toxic to the ovaries, especially in high doses. Full body and pelvic radiation are most likely to bring on menopause, and the older you are at the time of treatment, the more likely you are to go through early menopause as a result.

Ovary Removal: When you have both ovaries surgically removed, menopausal symptoms will occur immediately, your period will stop, and hormone levels will drop immediately.

Uterus Removal: If you undergo a hysterectomy, your risk of developing early menopause almost doubles. This was found in a Duke University study that confirmed that 14.8% of women who had hysterectomies went through menopause during the study, compared to 8% of women who didn't have surgery.

Various Health Conditions: Certain auto-immune diseases like thyroid and rheumatoid arthritis may cause the body's auto-immune system to attack the ovaries, causing them to stop making sufficient amounts of hormones. HIV and AIDS, when it is not controlled properly, may also lead to early menopause, and the same goes for women who have missing chromosomes and chronic fatigue syndrome (ME/CFS).

TIMELINE OF TRANSITION

Phases Explained: Perimenopause to Postmenopause

While the moment of menopause, as we define it, refers to a specific day in your life, as you will see below, the process or metamorphosis of menopause takes years to complete. In the west, we have broken down the menopause process into different phases, each with certain defining characteristics. Let's look at these phases one by one.

Perimenopause

Perimenopause marks the prelude to the main event that is menopause, as your body begins to rehearse the changes between 2-8 years before your last period. 'Peri,' by the way, means 'near' or 'around,' so directly translated, perimenopause means 'around the time of menopause.' As I mentioned, this phase usually starts in the late 30s to early 40s for Western women. At this time, you may notice some subtle changes in your body brought on by hormonal changes.

Here are some of the most common signs of perimenopause :

- Irregular periods,

- Increase in PMS symptoms,
- Heavy menstrual bleeding, also called menstrual flooding,
- Decreased sex drive or libido,
- Night sweats and hot flashes.

Menopause

What if I told you that the term 'Menopause' actually refers to only one day in your life? We talk a lot about menopause and use the word pretty loosely, but in reality, 'menopause' is defined as being one specific day in your life, that day being the 365th day following the last day of your last period.

This means, of course, that you can only know retrospectively when you have reached menopause, and the reason that this day is medically relevant is that at that point, your body no longer produces sufficient estrogen to be able to support a menstrual cycle. If you do have bleeding after that 365-day mark, this is something that you should have checked out.

Postmenopause

The day immediately after M-day, that magical 365-day milestone, you are considered to be post-menopausal. This is the time of new beginnings, and in survey after survey, post-menopausal women share how they are the most fulfilled and happiest they have ever been. They are relieved by not having periods anymore and not having to worry about falling pregnant.

My friend Marylin embodies this perfectly. Having mastered her own menopause, she has a sense of calm and control. She walks tall, having embraced the aging process. Her naturally gray hair looks like a silver halo, she is in great shape, she moves often and easily, and has a sense of serene calm about her. For her, menopause was an opportunity to connect more deeply with different aspects of herself, physically and spiritually.

Even if you are not having a Marylin-Menopause, and you are taking more strain, as your hormones become more stable over time, the associated symptoms, like migraines, PMS, and endometriosis, will also improve. You may still get some hot flashes for a couple of years, but even that will start to fade.

On the downside, the mucus membranes of your vagina will thin and dry over time, which may make sex uncomfortable, but there are simple ways to avoid that. There are, of course, other changes in your body at this time, and as time goes by, you may see your good cholesterol (HDL cholesterol) levels drop, and you may encounter issues with bone mass and muscle tone. While this may all sound like a hard pill to swallow, there are many ways to counter the effects of these changes and maintain a wholesome, healthy, fulfilling life. In the chapters following, I will give you a wide range of solutions and actionable strategies so that you can see what resonates with you, and you will be able to manage this life phase with clarity and grace.

Menopause vs. Aging:

Let's talk about the proverbial elephant in the room: AGING. This topic intertwines closely with the menopausal dance, yet it's a distinct performance in itself. Just as a dancer's repertoire spans various routines, understanding how menopause fits into the broader context of aging is important. We'll look at how menopause influences the aging process and how it stands apart as a unique stage in our lives.

Menopause, we know by now, is a normal life change. What is changing for our generation, and the next, is that our life expectancy is ever increasing, which means that today, we can expect to spend one-third or more of our lives in the post-menopausal phase. For this reason, it is becoming more and more important to understand the physiology of menopause and the effects it has on aging and our health into our later years.

The undeniable truth is that, as a general rule, menopause accelerates biological aging; in fact, it can increase cellular aging by 6%, on average.

What causes this accelerated aging? The main culprit seems to be insomnia, and anyone who has been through 'the change' will quickly tell you that sleepless nights are a close companion during perimenopause and menopause; whether your sleep is restless or you are struggling to fall asleep, the outcome is that your daily functioning will be affected and you will age faster, according to a study published in the journal Biological Psychiatry. [3]

This is not great news for any of us. Still, again, there are many natural ways to improve sleep, which we will look at later in this book. If you can view this as an opportunity to learn to regulate yourself better, you can come out better on the other end of this disruptive process.

GLOBAL GLIMPSE

As I was doing my early research about menopause, I started wondering how women from other places in the world, where they may not have all the medical facilities, tests, and medications have coped with menopause. I started looking into this and what I found delighted and surprised me. Let's have a look at how others embrace the dance of menopause.

It seems like Western women have a much harder time during menopause than most of our counterparts across the globe. Sure, there are many valid biological explanations for this but we have to also look at the broader picture and consider how our social and cultural attitudes affect the severity of our symptoms.

Cultural Interpretations and Responses

In patriarchal culture, as is prevalent in much of the world still, older women very often face negative stereotypes and criticism and are perceived and labeled as being unattractive, unhappy, and even useless. Where do these labels come from? Well, it really is extremely pervasive, and we see these messages, sometimes subtly and often not so subtly, in the media, in advertising, in the workplace, and even within our families. The message is loud and clear: Menopausal women should step aside!

This approach stands in stark contrast to that of many other cultures that have long recognized the value of menopause. Let's start by looking at a prime example: Japan, where there was no word for "hot flash" until they recently coined new terms like *"hotto furasshur"* (hot flash) and *"horumon baransu"* (hormone balance). Interestingly, only about a quarter of Japanese women ever report experiencing hot flashes, and shoulder stiffness is a more common menopause symptom in Japan.

Let's take it a little further and look at the Japanese word for menopause, "Konenki," which means "renewal and regeneration." Doesn't this point to a much more positive outlook than the English word, which points simply and quite harshly to the end of your monthly bleeding?

In cultures like Kaliai, Papua New Guinea, Native Americans, subcontinental Indians, and northern Sudan, menopause comes without troublesome symptoms. It also brings women more social power and respect, and women welcome the end of their childbearing years.

Some Mayan women seem to not have any traditional menopausal symptoms, which may be attributed to their lower body weight, their clean diet, or the possibility that in their culture it is not acceptable to speak about menopause. On an objective level, it has been found that Mayan women, as well as Japanese women, suffer from osteoporosis much less despite the fact that they also have lower estrogen as well as lower bone mineral density.

Could this be attributed to the fact that these Mayan have a more positive outlook on menopause and they are generally more optimistic about life after menopause? Because they see it as coming into freedom and status. Perhaps their cruising through menopause is the result of a slower life and their cultural outlook on menopause as a passage to wisdom and spiritual leadership.

You see, how we perceive menopause culturally can significantly impact our individual experiences. For example, Greek peasant women who expect hot flashes tend to experience more of them, and rural women in Iran who equate their value with their fertility have more negative feelings around menopause than their urban counterparts.

Thankfully, things are changing, and increasingly, even American women are coming to realize that menopause can indeed be a spiritually and personally transformative time and can bring us into the most powerful versions of ourselves. More and more, women over 50 are thriving and doing so publicly, including in the arenas of entertainment and politics.

Ancient Wisdom: How ancestral women coped

Menopause is not a new thing and even ancient Greeks had an awareness of this phenomenon. In fact the word 'menopause' comes from the Greek: 'men,' meaning 'month' like 'moon'; and 'pausis' from 'pauein,' which means 'to stop or to cease'. So, menopause refers to the time when a woman's monthly cycle comes to an end.

In ancient Greece, however, menopause wasn't paid much attention to, partially because women seldom lived past the age of 34, and also, women were only valued for their ability to bear children, so not much study was dedicated to their well-being post their fertile years.

Up until the 18th century, menopause was viewed as a natural part of the cycle of a woman's life, and it was only after that, that doctors started viewing it as a state of disease, leading to the development and use of a variety of strange and even dangerous therapies to be developed to treat menopause.

In the Victorian era, menopausal women were believed to be crazy, and were diagnosed with something called 'climacteric insanity', sometimes they were even locked up in asylums. It was quite normal at that time to remove the ovaries of menopausal women, hoping that would make them more compliant and hard working.

Modern vs. Traditional: Comparing approaches

In some cultures, for example the Maori in New Zealand and the Iroquois Indians, women that have gone through menopause are seen as spiritual elders and community leaders, while in traditional shamanic cultures it is believed that going through this change gives women shamanic and healing powers.

The Mayans and Cree women of Canada see menstrual blood as "wise blood," and because post-menopausal women retain this "wise blood," they become spiritual leaders, like priestesses and healers. Quite rightfully, these women are then given leadership roles because they have the capacity to support the community because they no longer have a responsibility to birth and rear their own infants. It's easy to see how an approach like this can benefit the overall population and success of the community, leading to the placement of older women at the center of societies in many cultures.

In our Western societies, unfortunately, there is not much value placed on the wisdom and spiritual growth that a woman gains from the transition into menopause, and in our youth-obsessed culture, aging women are often told, in no uncertain terms, to stand aside. It is this culture that also leads women like my friend Anna, I mentioned earlier, to feel that once they can no longer reproduce, she has no more value in society.

But where did this shift happen, and why? To answer this question, all we have to do is to take a quick look at the 'father of psychology', Sigmund Freud, and his theory of human development that essentially emphasizes that a woman's value relates to our ability to bear children, and becomes plain to see how this distorted view has immensely influenced the American view of women in menopause.

The truth is, thankfully, that more and more women worldwide are starting to see post-menopause as a time of feeling within themselves, and they feel a new surge of life-force energy, quite contrary to the jaded Freudian perspective.

I suggest embracing the empowering concept of the 'grandmother hypothesis.' It suggests that your menopausal phase is not just a personal transition but a vital contribution to the greater tapestry of life. By nurturing and supporting your 'grandchildren' (which may be human blood-related children or projects that uplift the youth in your community) and supporting your community, you play a pivotal role in shaping the future and strengthening your people's survival. Recognizing the wisdom you possess as a menopausal woman can lead to a profound self-celebration and a much more fulfilling life journey.

With all this being said, let's now look at the actual symptoms you may expect to experience during your menopausal period.

2
SYMPTOM SPECTRUM - FROM MILD TO WILD

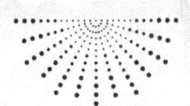

As of 2020, nearly half of women around the globe were unaware of perimenopause and were surprised when it started. Imagine the uncertainty and turmoil you go through when your body starts changing inexplicably without having any idea that you are in perimenopause. Sudden hot flashes, mood swings, emotional changes, weight gain… imagine the inner turmoil as you blame yourself and tell yourself that you are doing something wrong, while in reality, a process is unfolding over which you do not have control. [1]

How can you prepare yourself and avoid this from happening to you? Well, the first step is to know the symptoms so that, when it happens to you, you will understand what is going on, and you will be able to take charge and stay in the driver's seat of your life's journey. Sure, it won't make the symptoms go away; you will go through rocky phases and face a few crazy obstacles, but at least you will know to put your vehicle into a 4-wheel drive and brace yourself for the adventure ahead.

What follows is a simple summary of the most common symptoms of menopause in the words of real women. You should keep in mind that different women experience the symptoms in different ways. One woman may have almost no symptoms, while another may find herself crippled by the overwhelming amount of symptoms she has. Each of us has our own story, blueprint, and unique experiences.

THE BIG 7: USUAL SUSPECTS OF MENOPAUSE

1. **Hot Flashes and Night Sweats**

Many of us have experienced a hot flash at one point or another. That sudden feeling of warmth, starting in your chest and creeping up to your neck and your face, sometimes even accompanied by the reddening of your skin. It's like blushing or that hot-under-the-collar feeling when something makes you angry, or you get a sudden adrenaline rush through your body. Sometimes, you even get it when you eat your favorite hot curry or chili burger.

It's one thing to have these hot flashes happen when you are awake and can identify a logical reason for it, but imagine the overwhelm of having hot flashes suddenly occurring at night, with no obvious cause, and having them keep you up, even though you need your 8 hours of sleep. That, dear reader, is the reality of the notorious menopausal hot flashes. They are so notorious because hot flashes happen to be the most common symptom of menopause. So, if you are suddenly experiencing inexplicable surges of heat through your body, especially at night…consider that this may be the first sign of your menopause.

Oh, did I mention these flashes do not dance solo? They bring a few good friends, like rapid heartbeat, perspiration, anxiety, and a cold feeling, as they leave the party, which usually takes 2-5 minutes. Sounds like fun? Not really, right? Let's look at some quick ways to deal with and minimize these not-so-hot companions who will be with you for around seven years if you are like most Western women:

- Don't smoke; women who smoke tend to get more hot flashes;
- Lose the extra pounds, as high BMI is associated with more hot flashes;
- Keep cool - make sure you can remove layers as you get warm, drink cold water, and buy yourself a pocket fan to have handy at all times;
- Ditch the spices, caffeine, and alcohol;
- Manage your stress, meditate, and mind your breathing (more about this in Chapter 5)

But what causes this? Here's the thing: no one knows for sure, but the experts have a theory that lower estrogen levels make you more sensitive to changes in your body temperature. This is not very helpful, I know, and hopefully, over the next few years, science will be able to figure out the culprit so we can manage this symptom better.

Let's meet Linda, a 50-year-old freelance graphic designer, who began experiencing the tumultuous waves of menopausal hot flashes. Rather than let it dampen her spirit, Linda embraced this new phase with creativity and resilience.

In her home studio, where she spent hours designing, Linda started to keep a small, stylish fan, which not only provided relief during hot flashes but also became a quirky accessory on her desk. She adapted her wardrobe to chic, breathable fabrics, allowing her to stay comfortable and fashionable.

Linda also found support and understanding from her family. Her partner, aware of her night sweats, surprised her with cooling bed sheets, making their nights more comfortable. Her teenage daughter, inspired by Linda's openness about menopause, began a school project on women's health, further strengthening their bond.

What made Linda's journey through menopause unique was her ability to infuse her experience with her artistic flair. She even started a blog, sharing her menopausal experiences and creative solutions with a growing audience of women going through similar challenges. Linda's story is a testament to facing life's transitions with grace, creativity, and the loving support of family.

2. **Mood Swings and Emotional Changes**

"When we wake up, I never know what version of my wife will wake up next to me. After 20 years, I feel I should, but the mood swings are very unpredictable. I have had to learn to roll with the punches."

This is a comment from one of my friend's husbands, and I have heard this being echoed by several men in my circle. So, what does this mean? How intense are these so-called 'mood swings,' and what causes them?

Perhaps you are one of the lucky few who will not experience this. Otherwise, here's what you can expect: You will be cranky and angry. As your hormone levels fluctuate, you will feel irritable, often for no apparent external reason; the occasional (or not-so-occasional) bout of anger might overtake you, and you will often feel like you are on an emotional rollercoaster and every now and then, this rollercoaster seems to take you to Sad-Town. Melancholy Lane could become your second home some days.

As this is all happening, try to remember that while all this may feel so very real, it can be explained by the dips in hormone levels that come and go.

Just as you think that's all you can manage, you realize that you are forgetting things and have trouble concentrating: these memory lapses and difficulties with focus leaves you frustrated and confused. 'What on earth is going on with me?' seemed to be the question I asked myself at least a few times daily.

On top of all this, you are tired, fatigued, and just over it; you feel like you can sleep for days, except, as you will read about later, the sweet relief of a deep slumber seems out of reach.

As you can imagine, all of these changes can wreak havoc in your life, from your relationships to your job and everything in between. Don't feel too dismayed, though; we will be going through coping strategies in chapter 3!

3. Weight Gain and Metabolism Shifts

Here's the change that you probably fear more than any of the others. When I was younger, my perimenopausal friends kept telling me that after the age of 40, the pounds would pile on. I refused to believe them, arrogantly thinking this wouldn't ever happen to me. I've always been one of those who can take control easily by cutting down on carbs and working out a little. Was I in for a surprise!

So, why does this happen? There are several contributing factors to menopausal weight gain. Some say that the weight gain is more likely due to aging and lifestyle changes than the menopausal hormone shifts itself.

Firstly, menopausal symptoms like hot flashes, poor sleep, and feeling low can make it harder to exercise and eat healthy food, and this inevitably will lead to weight gain. Add to this the fact that, around menopause, ordinary life pressures like work and taking care of aging parents make it difficult for many of us to put our health first.

As far as hormonal changes and weight go, the drop in estrogen levels post-menopause has a tendency to change our body shape, so fat gets stored more around your waist and not on your hips and thighs like it used to. In fact, postmenopausal women, on average, carry between 15 to 20% of their total body weight around their waists, compared to 5 to 8% before menopause.

If you are reading this and you are feeling the worries creeping in, rest assured that there are ways in which you can combat this weight gain, the usual, which we will look at in Chapter 6.

4. Sleep Disturbances/Insomnia

When you think of all the changes that are happening in your body during menopause, you might imagine that you will be tired and would want to sleep your days away until it is all over. Here's where it gets uncomfortable, though: you will probably not be able to get much shut-eye.

Leanne had been an average sleeper her whole life. Most nights she could fall asleep fairly easily and she would wake up feeling rested if not rejuvenated. As soon as she hit her mid-forties though, sleep became a distant memory. She would toss and turn and struggle with falling asleep if there was even the slightest disturbance. She woke up easily and she never felt rested anymore. Desperate, frustrated, and emotionally drained, she scoured the internet for solutions. It was the advice of a natural healer though that gave her the most insight: human beings sleep better (from young babies to old men) when you prepare the environment for sleep.

It felt like a light bulb moment! Leanne immediately changed her room to a cooler temperature (and changed her linen to pure cotton for good measure), she banned electronics from the bedroom (yes, all of them) and moved her alarm clock to the adjacent room (it helped her get up anyway). Watching series to fall asleep (which never really worked) was now a thing of the past and meditation was her sacred sleep ritual. So was an earlier dinner time. In a few weeks, while she still had a bit of difficulty now and then, her sleep situation was transformed.

So why is sleep during menopause such an issue? Well, firstly, the hot flashes will keep you up, and many of us wake up just before a hot flash occurs. Add to this that during menopause, a lot of women develop sleep apnea, and if that doesn't keep you up, depressive symptoms and anxiety are likely to keep the sleep fairy at bay. Luckily, regular exercise, medication, and alternative treatments like acupuncture can help relieve this and help you get the rest you need to get through this testing time, in the second part of this book - we will look at all these solutions.

5. Vaginal Dryness and Discomfort

Vaginal dryness, irritation, and pain during sexual intercourse is something that is quite prevalent during menopause and gets worse after menopause, and about 90% of women experience this! What's the culprit here? Something called Genitourinary Syndrome of Menopause (GSM), is a term used to describe menopausal symptoms brought on by plummeting estrogen.

After menopause, certain physical changes take place in your vagina, changes like tissue atrophy, in other words, the wasting or shrinking of the skin inside your vagina. I know this may sound absolutely terrifying, but again, there are ways to deal with this very efficiently. Here are some of those methods:

- Try applying more vaginal stimulation, whether that is through intercourse or self-stimulation;
- Use lubrication during intercourse;
- Hormone therapy is said to reduce vaginal dryness;
- Start a good skincare regime for your vaginal tissue;
- Avoid things that can irritate your vagina, like scented detergents, and personal hygiene products, including sanitary pads for urinary incontinence;
- Avoid synthetic material underwear for everyday use and rather opt for cotton underwear, leaving the synthetics for occasional use only.

6. Loss of Libido

"I used to love sex, and I was never the type to fake a headache or give my partner a cold shoulder, quite the opposite. Now, I don't even recognize this person who pretends to be asleep when my husband tries to get sexy, and who wears ugly tracksuits in an attempt to discourage his advances. What is happening to me?"

This is what I heard from my friend the other day, and this sentiment echoes the feelings of so many women going through menopause. Why is this?

During menopause, you go through many, many physical changes, as well as very deep and profound emotional changes. You will probably find yourself redefining your roles and your purpose, and this will inevitably put a strain on many of your existing relationships. Very few people like change, especially when that change sees a woman becoming more opinionated and firmer in her personal boundaries. Of course, this is not exactly a recipe for creating intimacy while all these changes are happening.

Again, decreased estrogen can also be blamed as it may see your sex drive decreasing. You may find that you don't get aroused easily, and then, of course, there is vaginal dryness, often leading to pain during intercourse. You can see how all this adds up, right?

Now add to this the simple fact that as we get older, our energy levels tend to decrease, we may start suffering from lowered body image (wrinkles seldom feel sexy), and we may pick up some health issues along the way, not to mention that our partners may start running into issues like erectile dysfunction.

In Chapter 4, we will look at this more closely and discuss how your lifestyle choices, mindset, and medication can help sort this out.

7. Memory Problems and Cognitive Changes

A friend recently commented, jokingly, about memory problems and cognitive changes being a perk of menopause because at least it helps you live in some kind of denial about the apparent falling apart of your life. While this may be an exaggeration meant to create humor, the part about menopausal memory loss being a thing is very true. About 2 out of three menopausal women run into trouble remembering things and complain of persistent brain fog.

If you suddenly find it difficult to make decisions, learn new things, or remember what day of the week it is or what you are doing in the kitchen, these may be signs of menopause. These changes are linked to the lowering of your reproductive hormones, especially estrogen, and the sleepless nights we talked about above certainly do not help - I do not know a single person who gets better at reasoning and remembering when they are tired.

As you age, your brain will have the natural tendency to slow down or deteriorate, and it is up to you to train your brain to stay fit and active. Whether you sign up for a university degree, do Sudoku or crossword puzzles, or finally take that course that you have been too scared to commit to, these will help you in the 'use it or lose it' scenario, plus it will make for more interesting conversations as you move into your middle age.

THE UNDERCOVER AGENTS OF MENOPAUSE

Bone Health and Osteoporosis

As you go through menopause, your risk of bone loss and osteoporosis increases due to lowered estrogen levels; with up to 20% of bone loss becoming a reality in this time, and for half of menopausal women developing osteoporosis, it makes sense to take note of and gain a deeper understanding of this condition. So, what exactly is osteoporosis? It is defined as a progressive condition where your bones become structurally weak and, therefore, become prone to fracturing, leading to pain and lowered mobility.

Thankfully, treatment for osteoporosis can be effective at any age; for many older people, while early intervention is always best, it is never too late to start taking care of your bones!

How can you help prevent osteoporosis? Here are some tips:

- Make sure you get enough Vitamin D; the sun is (sort of) your friend, and Vitamin D will help you absorb calcium better;
- On that point, increase your calcium intake, calcium is crucial for bone health, and a lack thereof leads to weakened bones and a higher risk of fractures;
- If you follow a vegan or vegetarian diet, make sure you get all the nutrients you need as these diets may impact bone

health negatively and are associated with lower bone mineral density (BMD).

Skin and Hair Changes

About half of us will develop skin issues during menopause due to the lowering production of estrogen, progesterone, and testosterone, as well as the increase in our bodies' production of cortisol.

The skin issues I am talking about range from age spots to dry skin, acne, sagging skin, wrinkles, large pores, unwanted facial hair, an increased risk of skin cancer, and thinning skin.

How do you combat this?

- Use a daily SPF 30 or higher skin lotion;
- Make sure you do regular skin cancer screenings with a dermatologist;
- Practice skin self-exams and consult a dermatologist for age spot treatments;
- Stay hydrated, stop smoking if you are still doing that, and watch your alcohol intake;
- Use a mild cleanser, and moisturize with hyaluronic acid or glycerin;
- See a dermatologist if your skin is extremely dry;
- Consider laser hair removal or lotions meant for unwanted facial hair;
- Fight the face sagging and wrinkling effects of collagen with sun protection and a retinol or peptide facial product;
- Establish an anti-acne skincare routine with gentle treatments like salicylic acid cleansers;
- Your skin may become more sensitive during menopause, and you may get more rashes, so use a fragrance-free moisturizer to help with this.

Something that I never realized before going through it myself is that hormones, like estrogen and progesterone, can even impact our hair during perimenopause and postmenopause. One of the first things you may notice is that your hair may start thinning because declining estrogen disrupts the balance with dihydrotestosterone.

You may also start noticing dry, dull strands of hair; this results from reduced sebum production, and your scalp can become more sensitive. Dry scale causes tiny cracks in your skin, exposing the scalp to irritants and inflammation.

If you are anything like me, a good hair day is often an indication that you will have a good day, while a bad hair day can have the opposite effect. So, how can we manage these changes to our hair while going through menopause?

There are Hormone Replacement (HR) options that can alleviate these symptoms; this is something your doctor can discuss with you. If you are not quite ready for that step, you can stimulate hair growth using topical minoxidil, encourage growth with natural hair oils like jojoba, castor, peppermint, or you can try LED therapy for follicular stimulation.

Also make sure you take care of your scalp by cleansing, stimulating, and moisturizing it carefully. Thickening shampoos with biotin and proteins can help your hair feel fuller, and smoothing treatments or salon keratin treatments can make it more manageable.

Irregular Menstruation

Irregular menstruation is one of the most common symptoms of perimenopause, and very few women get away from that during their menopausal years. It is, as most menopause symptoms are, caused by fluctuating and declining hormone levels; menopause disrupts the regulation of periods by estrogen and progesterone hormones, leading to erratic oscillations and varied menstrual patterns.

Irregular periods are often the first sign of perimenopause, and they start between two to ten years before menopause.

As you know already, our cycles are all different, and most of us have irregular periods at some point in our lives, and while the occasional cycle variances does not automatically mean you are in menopause, if you are over 40, and you are experiencing this somewhat regularly, be aware that you may be in perimenopause. It also helps to know that spotting in between irregular periods is normal during menopause, and while you may sometimes not have a period for months, do remember that while fertility does decline during menopause, you can still fall pregnant.

The usual lifestyle culprits: stress, dietary changes, and underlying health problems can be at the trigger point of irregular periods, and if it carries on beyond a few months, have it checked out; as I always say, rather safe than sorry when it comes to your health!

As we will explore in depth later in this book, changes to your diet, reducing stress, getting enough sleep, and smoking less (or preferably quitting altogether) can help regulate your period again.

Anxiety and Depression

This is a major symptom that causes havoc in our lives as we go through menopause, and we have already touched on this. In Chapter 3, we will take a deep look into the psyche during this transition phase. Rest assured that I will offer you many helpful tips and remedies that will help you through this.

Heart Health

Up until menopause, we women actually have a lower risk of heart disease than men, but as estrogen levels decrease during perimenopause, our risk for heart disease increases, our heart disease risk surpassing that of men. Interestingly, heart disease is the number one health risk for menopausal women.

Based on the 1980s-1990s studies, HRTs were thought to lower the risk of heart disease in menopausal women, but a 2002 study contradicted that assumption and also raised concerns about the potential risks of HRTs. It is thought that the timing of estrogen treatment and the interaction with progestin caused the conflicting results and today HRT is not clinically recommended for preventing heart disease.

Digestive Problems

When we go into menopause, most women tend to experience more gastrointestinal (GI) symptoms, like abdominal pain, discomfort, and bloating, than before menopause.

According to a study [2] of 18 research papers from 1980 to 2008 scrutinizing the link between menopause and gastrointestinal issues, it was found that visceral pain sensitivity is significantly higher during menstruation in women with IBS, suggesting that there may be a connection between hormonal changes and symptom severity.

To combat gastrointestinal issues, you can tailor certain habits and remedies. For example, make sure you chew food thoroughly to initiate effective digestion, thereby reducing strain on your stomach. You can also make sure you have regular eating times, without interference, so your energy is fully focused on digesting the food you consumed in that eating time. This also allows you to be mindful about eating foods that you can digest easily, to lessen strain on the digestive system.

Lastly, stay hydrated and avoid caffeine, alcohol, and refined sugar to reduce strain on both the digestion and the nervous system, and you can manage this pesky symptom with ease.

Joint Pain and Muscle Aches

Arthralgia is a complex sounding word to explain a simple concept: Joint pain and muscle aches. Women in menopause tend to report this more, and this is, like many other symptoms we have looked at, linked to declining estrogen levels. Keep in mind that abruptly stopping hormone replacement therapy or using aromatase inhibitors can also cause this condition.

Studies show a complex connection between sex hormones, immune cells, and cartilage cells (chondrocytes), but we don't understand a lot about it yet, so I will offer you some practical ways to deal with this, instead of trying to understand something that science is still figuring out.

Firstly, HRT can help, and so can weight loss, and regular exercise. Pain relievers may alleviate joint pain, particularly if you have underlying osteoarthritis. You can also look at other lifestyle related factors like fatigue, poor sleep, sexual problems, and depression, as indication of your overall well-being because the better your overall health, the better you will be able to cope with this.

Headaches and Migraines

During our different life stages, puberty, pregnancy, menopause, and hormone medications, our hormone levels change. I remember getting my first and really intense migraines as I went into puberty, and throughout my life, I encountered hormone-related migraines and headaches from time to time. What is the reason for this?

You guessed it: It's the estrogen again; when estrogen withdraws from your body, it can trigger migraines. Progesterone also has an effect on migraines, although the reason for the link is somewhat unclear.

Managing migraines tied to hormonal changes is difficult and usually medications and adjustments to hormone levels is recommended.

In terms of more holistic and natural approaches, you can look at improving your sleep hygiene, taking it easy on the caffeine, reducing stress, and getting more exercise.

Bladder Health

During menopause, as your estrogen decreases, you may start experiencing urogenital atrophy (muscle loss) – and a decline in vaginal and urinary tract health. Your bladder and your urethra can weaken as well, disrupting your control over urinary functions.

In addition to this, the reduced estrogen in your body can change the acidity in your vulva and vagina, inviting unwanted infections by bacteria or yeast.

Depending on your individual experience, these may be minor inconveniences or you may find them so stressful that it leads to emotional distress. The challenge here is that, unlike hot flashes, urogenital atrophy symptoms worsen with age instead of dissipating.

So, how do you know that this is happening? If you find that laughing, coughing, or sudden movements cause leaks, or you have sudden, strong urges to urinate and make more frequent trips to the bathroom and you suddenly wake up several times each night to urinate, these are all telltale signs.

What are the treatment options? HRT, to increase estrogen, along with local applications of estrogen like creams, tablets, or rings may help with symptoms while lifestyle changes like reducing caffeine, weight management, and pelvic floor exercises can help with the underlying causes.

Eye Changes

Finding yourself squinting more to see property or battling to see things that are far away? During menopause, your declining estrogen levels can also affect your eyesight and eye health due to pressure fluctuations. Even your eye shape can change slightly and you may find that your contact lenses don't even fit properly anymore.

Your eyes can also start feeling drier, for the same reason you are experiencing vaginal dryness: your mucus membranes are changing or, on the other extreme, your eyes may become watery. Menopause may also increase the risk of serious eye conditions like glaucoma and cataracts.

What to do about it: Firstly, reduce screen time if you can, have regular eye tests done, take menopause support supplements (more about this later), try natural remedies like Sea Buckthorn Oil, and use eye drops.

On the nutrition side, try to eat more brightly colored foods rich in lutein, zeaxanthin, and vitamin A like kale, spinach, and broccoli in your diet. Additionally, supplement with 15 mg zinc daily and, of course, stay hydrated with 1.5 liters daily.

SEVERITY AND SPAN OF SYMPTOMS

Every woman experiences menopause differently, and while some of us may not experience any noticeable symptoms, others may feel as if they are experiencing every one of them. For some, menopause goes by in a heartbeat, and others battle for years and years. So, why the differences?

Here are some factors that play a role, and by empowering yourself with this knowledge, you may be able to reduce your symptoms and the longevity thereof:

Genetic Factors like genetic predisposition and family history can influence how you experience menopause. This being said, it also may not. A good friend of mine whose mother has almost no menopause symptoms is going through a lengthy, full-blown menopause experience herself, for example.

Hormonal variability, meaning the rate and extent of estrogen and progesterone, affects the onset and intensity of symptoms.

Health and lifestyle, like pre-existing medical conditions, diet, exercise, and overall health, impact your symptoms.

Reproductive histories, like the number of pregnancies and childbirth experiences, may cause different hormonal profiles and, therefore, different experiences.

Surgical menopause vs. natural menopause has an effect since removal of your ovaries may cause more sudden and intense symptoms because of the abrupt decline in hormone levels.

Psychological factors like stress, mental health, and attitude toward menopause have an effect and women with a positive mindset may cope better with symptoms.

Ethnic and cultural differences can significantly shape how symptoms are perceived.

Body composition, meaning your body fat distribution can have an impact on estrogen levels: if you have a higher fat percentage, onset of your symptoms may be more gradual.

Individual sensitivity to hormonal changes can also impact how you perceive or experience your own symptoms.

Now that we have looked at all the major symptoms broadly, let's zoom in on the ones that cause the most distress to us, starting with the emotional havoc that menopause may cause.

3
NAVIGATE THE EMOTIONAL ROLLERCOASTER

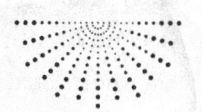

I remember a family lunch a few years ago where I saw first-hand the effect that menopause can have on women's emotions. My mother-in-law, a woman who has generally always been soft-spoken and even-tempered, was getting things ready for the family lunch. The family was milling about as usual, chatting here and there and, in general, just congregating.

For what seemed to us at the time as a result of no particular reason, my mother-in-law suddenly flew into a fit of rage and started yelling at all and sundry about the family lunch. Her words may have been about nobody helping her or feeling underappreciated (both of which were quite true at that moment, much to our collective shame), but the scale of her reaction made us realize quite quickly that there was more going on than what we were aware of.

Quietly, we each grabbed something from the kitchen and headed outside to the table, leaving my father-in-law to pick up the pieces. To our amazement, both came outside after just a few short minutes, and sat us down for a frank conversation. My mother-in-law explained that she was currently going through menopause and that she was experiencing extremely abrupt and severe mood swings. To this day, I am grateful and proud that she did not apologize for what was happening to her but rather explained it to us, and with the support of my father-in-law, she laid out some information that helped us all navigate it in the years to come.

I found out many years later that those quiet moments that my father-in-law spent with her in the kitchen that day was him reassuring her, repeating phrases and breathing exercises that they had looked up and practiced together. I can say without a doubt that having those tools at hand, armed with information and a supportive spouse, is the number one reason why my mother-in-law handled menopause so gracefully - and without losing her mind even if she did still endure mood swings and a whole host of other symptoms.

MAP THE EMOTIONAL TERRAIN

Having insight into the nature of menopause allows us to better prepare for it. We have explored the physicality of it and all the associated symptoms, but what about the emotional ups and downs you are bound to experience? Emotional and psychological shifts are to be expected during this phase of your life, but how do you navigate them and prepare yourself to the best of your ability to ensure mental wellness? In this chapter, we will delve a little deeper into the changes you can expect and the actionable strategies you can implement along the way. Let us take the time now to understand and manage the full spectrum of emotions that menopause can affect and what you can do about it.

Understand Emotional Shifts

Our first step is to come to grips with the emotional shifts that are taking place. Let's get our facts straight and investigate what we are actually dealing with.

The Hormone-Mood Connection

Your mood is largely determined by the hormonal balances in your body. Primarily, Dopamine (which plays a crucial role in the brain's pleasure and reward centers) and Serotonin (the body's "happy hormone") are the essential contributing hormones to your emotional state. An imbalance can lead to feelings of depression or anxiety - mood disorders aggravated by the destabilization of your hormones. Lower estrogen levels caused by menopause and the associated effects also contribute negatively to the overall impact on your mood.

How long does menopause affect mental and emotional well-being?

The answer to this question will be different for every woman because the duration of menopause (perimenopause all the way through to postmenopause) is different for every woman. The reality is that as long as your body is undergoing the effects of menopause, it may affect your emotional and mental well-being. Since your hormones play such a crucial role in your mental and emotional state, it stands to reason that as long as these are unbalanced and changing, you will experience the effects on your well-being. For most women, this period can last anywhere from 7 to 14 years.

Can menopause affect my self-image and self-esteem?

For most women, the answer is yes. Menopause can affect your feelings of confidence and self-identity in tremendous ways and requires a good dose of inner work to combat. Reminding yourself of your intrinsic value - not tied to youth or reproductive ability -

is incredibly important during menopause. Remember that you are worth so much more than the sum of your parts and that menopause, albeit overwhelming at times, is temporary.

Why do I feel a sense of loss or grief during menopause?

Feelings of grief and loss are completely natural during menopause. These feelings are both rational and common during any transition in our lives though we seldom have the tools with which to express it. Most of us associate grieving with the loss of a loved one, but losing an older version of yourself can be just as traumatic. The potential for grief, or a deep sense of sadness, is present during every major life change or upheaval, and menopause is no different.

Why am I experiencing irritability or bouts of rage?

Menopausal rage is real - and it can be mitigated - however it is important to know why it is happening in the first place. Here again, we have hormones to thank: the constant fluctuations in your estrogen, progesterone, and the lower levels of serotonin can cause irritability, depression, and often sudden, difficult-to-control bouts of rage. Remember, too, that you may be dealing with fatigue, sleep issues, anxiety, hot flashes, and more, all of which can create tension and feelings of rage.

Beyond Hormones: External Stressors and Changes

Another thing to remember about your emotional and mental well-being during menopause is the effect it can have on your capacity to deal with external stress. Life happens, and so does work stress (aggravated by feelings of mental fogginess or physical discomfort), relationship stress (aggravated by feelings of low self-esteem, low sex drive, and general irritability), and not mention other major life events such as death, divorce, moving, or other major transitions.

Grief and Acceptance: Mourning reproductive ability

As we have discussed above, feelings of grief during menopause are completely natural and normal. Many women mourn the loss of their reproductive ability - and for a wide spectrum of reasons. For some, it is the sense of lost opportunity, perhaps even that they may have wanted to have (more) children. For others, and this isn't mutually exclusive from wanting to bear children, it could be the fact that they have lost control over their reproductive ability. Sometimes, it is tied in with the loss of youth, the fear of age and decline, or even the uncertainty that comes with change. For most women however, menopause is an amazing period of acceptance as well - a time to embrace a new season of your life. Allow yourself to mourn but seek help if it turns into depression.

Faye, a holistic healer that I had the pleasure of working with during my menopause journey, gave me some insight into the transitions that women face. At every stage of change, we experience the duality of excitement about the new season of our life, as well as the grief and sadness associated with leaving a stage we have grown accustomed to. Of course, she provided this insight through the lens of growth - how, without discomfort and loss, we could never achieve change and we would only experience stasis - remaining the same without ever having the ability to evolve. Since we know that life demands this change whether we like it or not, we can better prepare ourselves for the upheaval it represents. That does not mean that it won't affect our emotions or create feelings of grief.

It is our responsibility (towards ourselves as well as our loved ones and others around us) to take on the mantle of change and forge our path ahead with both intention and gusto or "Purpose and Passion" as Faye called it. We have an amazing ability to adapt both as women and as human beings - in other words it is in our nature to be able to change. Menopause is one of the biggest changes you might experience in your life and it is both extremely personal and, as we saw in chapter 1, it is completely universal in nature. Every single woman will go through menopause in her life and every single woman will have feelings about it. Faye left me with this amazing truth: "To mourn who you once were is natural, necessary, and noteworthy, but it demands that you also accept your new life and move from mourning to celebration." She also made the point, however, of explaining how much easier said than done this can be and that there are emotional dangers we need to be aware of during the process.

DEPRESSION AND MENOPAUSE

Deciphering Symptoms: Menopause or Depression? How do I differentiate?

Depression and menopause are often mistaken for the other since the symptoms are so similar. Many women are actually misdiagnosed as having depression when, in reality, they have simply started their journey into menopause and need support for their changing hormones. Fatigue, weight change, sleep issues, low sex drive, and poor concentration are all symptoms of both menopause and clinical depression - so how do you tell the difference? If these feelings suddenly begin in your early 40's then menopause is the most likely culprit. Menopausal depression also fluctuates quite a lot, and you are more prone to experiencing it if you have also suffered from PMS. Clinical depression is a much deeper sadness - far more intense and lasting for much longer without reprieve. Often coupled with feelings of hopelessness, worthlessness, and helplessness, clinical depression can also lead to suicidal thoughts or self-harm. If you or someone you know is experiencing suicidal thoughts or thoughts of self-harm, please contact your healthcare provider immediately. Never diminish or dismiss these feelings - they are valid, important, and completely normal. It is always better to be safe and to get the support you need.

The Risk Factors and Triggers

As mentioned above, you may be more at risk for menopausal depression if you have suffered from extreme bouts of PMS during your life. The major risk factors for developing menopausal depression or anxiety include: vasomotor symptoms (hot flashes, night sweats, etc.); previous history of a major depressive disorder; neuroticism; major changes at home or stressful life events; as well as low financial or educational status.

The lesser or minor risk factors for developing menopausal depression or anxiety include: a lack of social support; being single or divorced; having a negative perception of aging or of menopause, and, as mentioned before, a history of premenstrual syndrome (PMS) or premenstrual dysphoric disorder (PMDD) - the more severe extension of PMS that includes physical and behavioral symptoms which normally resolve at the onset of menstruation.

Seek Help: Therapy, Support Groups, and Medication

So how can you be proactive about menopausal depression and ensure that you have the best possible chance of making it through with your mental and emotional wellness intact? There are a number of different sources you can go to for help. Support groups are a big favorite because they allow you to relate to other women going through the same thing. Therapy is another great avenue, especially if you are naturally predisposed to depression without the onslaught of hormones currently raging in your body. For some women, medication is an amazing support that allows them to better handle the things life and menopause throws at them - simply by using medication to control and balance the hormonal changes that menopause induces.

ANXIETY'S GRIP

Recognizing Anxious Patterns

Closely related to depression, and in particular menopausal depression, is anxiety. Menopause can trigger not only intense feelings of sadness but also feelings of anxiousness, irritability, and a sense of being overwhelmed. How do you recognize when you are in the grips of anxious patterns? For starters, you may notice that your thoughts tend to be on the fatalistic side - adverse, extreme negatives that may or may not be founded in reality. Ask yourself what you are thinking about currently - what are you worried will happen, and what bad things do you expect to happen? Evaluate these thoughts, and you will see where your mind is struggling.

Hormonal Fluctuations and Anxiety

Another way to determine if your anxiety levels are being influenced by menopause is by taking stock of your other symptoms. Hormonal fluctuations cause physical effects in the body, and if these coincide with anxious feelings, then it is likely that you are suffering from menopausal anxiety. As we have seen, falling levels of estrogen, progesterone, and serotonin, can lead to feelings of depression and anxiety - that does not however mean that frequent, troublingly high levels of anxiety or panic attacks should be dismissed as normal. Use a healthy diet and supplement your hormonal fluctuations as recommended by your healthcare professional to ease and abate the symptoms of anxiety.

Breathing and Grounding Exercises

Another method for addressing anxiety during menopause is by using mindfulness to ease and calm your mental and emotional state. Breathing and grounding exercises are exceptionally useful to many women in this instance. Try using rhythmic breathing -

take slow measured inhales through the nose and paced, steady exhales out the mouth. Count to 4 for each inhale, hold for 4 counts, then exhale for 4 counts then increase all the way up to 8 as your breathing slows. Be mindful of your body and notice how it naturally relaxes. Use grounding techniques to notice tactile elements of your environment and focus briefly on each before moving on until you find yourself in a calm and peaceful state. There are a number of similar exercises you can use but these are the ones I have found to be the most useful when I feel overwhelmed and anxious.

EMPOWERMENT THROUGH SELF-CARE

Manage emotional high's with self-care

Now that we have looked at the effects of hormones on your mental and emotional state, and explored both depression and anxiety during menopause, let us switch focus to the gradual self-care tasks that can make you more resilient against these symptoms and improve your overall sense of wellness. If you are wondering whether there are natural remedies that can help you stabilize your mood, then you are in the right place - because yes, there are, and we are going to dive a little deeper into these remedies right here.

Mindfulness and Meditation

The Power of Presence

Presence, in other words the art of active being, requires both awareness and mindfulness. It requires you to pay attention to the present moment and allow it to consume your focus, all while still holding onto a sense of curiosity, openness, and non-judgement. Presence is a habit that can and should be cultivated in your life, especially when you are using mindfulness techniques to develop strategies for managing major life events such as menopause. Presence is powerful and can drastically transform the way your mind (read:brain) translates things throughout your body and spiritual being.

Simple Meditation Techniques for Beginners

There are entire volumes of meditation techniques that can be both useful for menopause and easy enough for even the ultimate novice to master. Here are some of my favorites:

The Hot Flash Deep Breath

First, you will want to sit in a straight-back chair with both of your feet on the floor. Rest your hands on the abdomen, and slowly inhale through the nose while counting to four. Feel your abdomen rise as you take your inhale and then hold that breath for a moment before a slow exhale to the count of four, breathing out the mouth and allowing the abdomen to slowly fall. Repeat this exercise as needed though I recommend a minimum of 15 minutes in the beginning and end of the day (or as a hot flash arises).

The MenoPAUSE Body Scan

Find a quiet place where you will feel totally at ease with your eyes closed. Take a few deep breaths and 'tune in' to your body. Starting at the head and moving down to your toes, become aware of every sensation including tightness, pain, temperature, pressure, and so on. Think of this as a quick diagnostic to ensure that you are fully aware of what your body needs and use it to adapt your self-care tasks.

The Love and Kindness Meditation

Sit comfortable in a quiet space and place your hand lightly on your chest. Say kind phrases to yourself OUT LOUD, especially when you feel particularly out of balance with what you are saying. Tell yourself that you can and will make it through this phase of your life; remind yourself that you deserve happiness and peace; make kind wishes towards yourself. It might help to envision people that care about you saying these things. It may also help to picture the things that you would want to say to someone you care about in this situation.

Guided Imagery and Visualization

There are some wonderful visualization and guided imagery exercises out there for managing menopause. The practice involves the seemingly simple act of visualizing an object, scene, or even an event that you associate with a sense of calmness or joy. You will need to close your eyes and picture your 'focus imagery' (the image you are using to focus), and then allow yourself to get lost in it for a few moments. Let your mind wander within the boundary of this visual alone, and once you feel grounded by the return to this state of calm or happiness, take a deep breath, return back to your present moment, and carry on with your life enjoying the added boost of mental and emotional clarity.

Helen, a high powered executive that was well regarded as a leader, known for being "a force to be reckoned with", found the idea of menopause to be completely crippling. When the first symptoms of menopause started, she felt a surge of panic and disconnection with her life. She sought the advice of her therapist on how to deal with the sudden onslaught of change and overwhelm, and she was advised to start mindfulness practices every day, in particular, using guided imagery and visualization exercises to get through difficult moments at work.

One afternoon, while running from one meeting to the next, she felt the onset of anxiety and panic as her body started experiencing physical symptoms again, specifically a rather intense hot flash. Instead of spiraling deeper into a state of emotional and mental dysregulation, she excused herself from the first few minutes of the meeting and went to sit in an empty office with a locked door to do a visualization exercise she had practiced with her therapist. Within just a few short minutes, she felt calm and in control again, ready to take on the rest of her day.

Journaling for Joy and Release

Expressive Writing Benefits

Research has proven that writing - and especially the physical act of putting pen to paper - offers benefits to both our mental health and physical well-being, such as faster healing and even an increase in immune system function. It helps dissipate stress, improve mental clarity, and provides you with the ability to make sense of your feelings and thoughts.

Menopause Mood Trackers

Speaking of gaining insight into your mental and emotional state, menopause mood trackers have become increasingly popular as a supplemental tool for managing and treating menopause. Not only does it allow you the personal insight that a mood tracker offers - forcing you to take mental and emotional stock at least once every day - but it gives you an overview of how your current treatment and management protocol is working. It helps you make changes to your menopause strategy in the areas where you need it most.

Here are my top three mood trackers:

- balance app - https://www.balance-menopause.com/balance-app/
- Mysysters - https://mysysters.com/
- Onstella - https://us.onstella.com/

Gratitude Practices

One of my favorite self-care techniques is that of owning my gratitude. I create moments of happiness and positive awareness around myself simply by taking the time to be grateful. It can be difficult at first to get started, especially if you are feeling physically, emotionally, and spiritually overwhelmed, but it is well worth it. Research has shown that gratitude is strongly and consistently associated with greater happiness.[1] It helps you feel more positive emotions, relish positive experiences, improve your health, and support building stronger relationships.

Here are some examples of gratitude practices I enjoy:

- Gratitude journaling (write down 3 things that you are grateful for every day);
- Write thank you notes, cards, or letters every week (even for mundane things);
- Finding the silver lining (I challenge myself to find it in every situation I face).

Creative Outlets

Art Therapy Basics

Art therapy is an amazing tool that allows therapists to guide their patients through understanding their emotions, through interpretation, expression, and even the resolution of thoughts and feelings. It is an expressive type of therapy that allows you to gain clarity by responding creatively to prompts and questions. Mediums for art therapy include painting, sculpture, drawing, collage - really any artistic form that suits you.

Dance and Movement: Body Expression

Another artistic form that can prove therapeutic during menopause is that of dance and movement. Using your body to express an idea, feeling, or simply to release pent up tension or emotion can be intensively rewarding. It's also great for your health! Dance and movement can warm up and soften ligaments, lower cholesterol, improve fitness, and boost your overall body composition (and for many your self-esteem too!).

Music and Mood Modulation

Studies [2] have found that music can help decrease the effects of menopause and the occurrence of depression in menopausal women. In fact, the effects are so significant that music has even been recommended as a non-pharmacological therapy option in nursing care. Music is a fantastic medium for mood modulation. Since music stimulates our body into producing feel-good hormones, it assists the body in better balancing hormonal changes and, therefore, in managing mood shifts.

How to balance self-care and my responsibilities towards the family?

Now for the thing that most women struggle with: balancing their own needs and taking care of themselves while still doing everything they need to do to look after their families (and work, social responsibilities, and so on). The thing is, unless you absolutely prioritize these self-care tasks, it may very easily become something you very much intend to do but never actually do.

The problem, of course, is that when you are not feeling your best - especially while you navigate something as monumental as menopause - it can be difficult, if not downright impossible, to take care of others. You need to put yourself first, this is the one time in your life, above all others, that you truly will not be able to get through unscathed without making yourself a priority.

Manage your time by always first creating and fiercely protecting time with yourself. Address unhealthy behaviors that your loved ones might have that could negatively affect your own wellness or your ability to prioritize your self-care. Delegate tasks where possible and seek external support to ensure that you maintain a good relationship with your own well-being. Above all else, take a break, remind yourself that your needs are paramount to the entire family's happiness and success, and create space to love yourself a little extra during menopause.

BUILD RESILIENCE AND EMOTIONAL MUSCLE

Positive Psychology Practices

Embracing Optimism: Seeing Beyond Symptoms

The art of optimism, and yes it is an art, is the backbone of creating a positive and empowering mindset that will help you survive and thrive this season of your life. As I have shared before, the practice of finding the silver lining, of focusing on the positive aspects of the situation instead of only the negative ones, can help you mitigate the feelings of depression, overwhelm, and frustration or stress that comes along with menopause. Remember that when you embrace optimism, you embrace a better reality for your inner and outer self.

Acts of Kindness: Boosting Feel-Good Hormones

Have you ever heard about the Helper's High? In the simplest terms, it refers to the release of dopamine that we get when we give unto others - random acts of kindness that trigger a chemical reaction in the body creating a sense of happiness and even euphoria in the giver. Now isn't that a handy way to create happy feelings within your own being while still being an awesome human to others?

The Value of Laughter and Humor

Laughter - and I'm talking about that feel good belly rumbling type of laughter - doesn't only make you feel good and draw you closer to the people around you but it actually improves your immune system, strengthens your ability to manage stress, and it reduces pain. Humor and laughter has the ability to help you manage your emotions better - it lightens your emotional and mental burden and it makes it easier to forgive, connect, focus, and create hope. If you want to make it through menopause, you need to prioritize a good sense of humor and laugh as much as possible.

Cognitive Behavioral Therapy (CBT) Insights

Reframing Thoughts: Turning Negatives into Neutrals

Cognitive behavioral therapy (CBT) allows us insight into why and how a perspective shift significantly affects our mental and emotional well-being. By better managing your thought patterns and behavior, you are able to actively intervene and change the way your body and mind see problems, symptoms, or experiences. To change a negative thought into a neutral one, you must first identify it. If you notice an inaccurate negative thought, try reframing it. Turn "I'm a failure" into "I made a mistake and I have the opportunity to learn from it so that I am better prepared next time."

The Value of Professional Guidance

When we think of CBT, we must always remember that it is, first and foremost, a therapy - it alters your perception of the world around you and requires meaningful inner work. It can be dangerous to try and rewrite your thought and behavior patterns without the proper support system and a trained professional to guide your process. Not only will your therapist be able to ask the right questions (at the right time) but they will act as a sounding board for the realizations you will have along the way. CBT is a talk- type therapy and that means, you need the right person to talk to.

Behavior Experiments: Testing Out New Reactions

Behavioral experiments (basically trying something in a new way to find a different result) are used to offer new information about a situation and can be quite powerful in effect. Many people who do the exercises are able to better evaluate and understand their behaviors and find they are now able to modify and improve their beliefs about an experience and its consequences. An example would be to change your bedtime routine, alter the clothing you wear or deodorants you use, or even to increase or change exercise levels and type - and then using this information to make stronger choices for your menopause strategy. You may find some things work far better for you than others and you can adapt accordingly.

Community, Connection, and Support

The Power of Shared Experience

The human experience has never been something to be undergone in isolation. As they say, "No man is an island" - and neither should we attempt to be. When we connect with others and share our experiences, it helps us understand in quite visceral fashion that we are not alone. Feeling heard, understood, and validated are some of the most important factors in creating a supportive space while you are navigating menopause. Without support, without feeling seen and valued, menopause becomes a difficult and lonely experience - oftentimes becoming more than a woman can bear.

Joining or Starting a Support Group

One of the best places to find this connection is by joining a support group. Support groups for menopause are not only excellent sources of comfort and connection, the communities that arise from these support groups offer you insight, emotional release, and quite frequently a wide range of additional resources that can prove incredibly helpful as you try to find answers and strategies for your personal menopause journey.

Remember also that there are great groups for your support system: partners often find it useful to gain insight about menopause from other partners going through similar experiences. It helps our partners gain insight, understanding, and actionable strategies for their own experience as well as learning how to better support us.

If you cannot find a menopause support group, you may think about starting one of your own. The key characteristics of a great support group are:

- Confidentiality
- Regular support sessions
- Succinct meetings
- Numerous useful, insightful, and readily available additional resources
- An open floor to encourage and welcome discussion that creates a safe space for everyone to be heard

Feel free to vary your format but remember to keep things factual and friendly.

Online Communities and Resources

To make things easier, I have created a short list of some great online communities, groups, and resources that could be helpful to you during your menopause journey:

Menopause Matters:

Facebook group - private group that offers support and resources during every phase of menopause https://www.facebook.com/groups/425415375251256/?mibextid=oMANbw

The Daisy Network:

Charity / Support Network - aimed specifically at women undergoing early menopause, offers live chats with specialists and more

https://www.daisynetwork.org/

Endocrine Society:

Online resource center - an invaluable resource center filled with printable personal path tools, downloadable literature and resources, support resources and more

https://www.endocrine.org/menopausemap/support-resources/index.html

Red Hot Mamas:

Support Group - a fantastic platform to start your support journey and join in the conversation that hosts a number of menopause topics

https://www.inspire.com/groups/red-hot-mamas-menopause/

Menopause and Me (US):

Online resource center - hosted by the North American Menopause Society, this resource platform offers access to annual meetings, publications, and more

https://www.menopause.org/for-women

Menopause and Me (UK):

Online resource center - filled with a wealth of information for every stage of menopause including podcasts, access to coffee catch ups, checklists, printable booklets, and more *https://www.menopauseandme.co.uk/en-gb*

Menopause can be an emotional rollercoaster - that does not mean you have to go through it alone. Any challenge that menopause might present can be overcome by using the right tools, strategies, and mindset. You are incredibly powerful and you have the ability to navigate this journey with both resilience and grace. Armed with the knowledge from this chapter, you are better equipped to handle your mental and emotional well-being as well as the fundamental dynamics of relationships that go along with it.

∼

4
SAILING SMOOTH - RELATIONSHIPS & MENOPAUSE

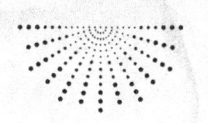

> *"...Mrignayani, the lover said,*
> *I need some distance.*
> *Shifting the focal length*
> *Gives great perspective.*
> *So he retreated,*
> *Into the vanishing point..."*

Menopause: A Poem - "My tongue has sharpened."

By Hema Gopinathan Sah

The other day, my friend, Nina, showed up at my door, sobbing tears of grief and guilt, desperate for a solution or at least some hope for the future. What caused this trouble to my typically temperate and joyful friend? She explained, after she managed to regulate her breathing and dry her eyes, that suddenly she had no desire to lay with her darling husband of 20 years. It's not that he changed or that she no longer loved him; she simply had no desire for sex. How is this possible? How could she sustain the relationship when every time he initiates intimacy, she shrinks away from his touch? She even spoke of wishing he would find a lover to take care of his 'physical needs,' and she would feel less pressured. How did this happen? Just a few months ago, this thought would not even occur to her and her husband making love to another person would sound like the worst thing in the world. What is going on?

INTIMATE INSIGHTS

The Libido Labyrinth - why has my libido decreased, and how can it affect my relationship?

During and after the period of menopause, many women see their libidos decreasing, they have orgasms less frequently, and they end up having coitus less often. The reason for this? Well, it is largely due to the physiological changes of menopause, the hormonal havoc we spoke about earlier, and it can also be attributed to mood changes, depression, and marital discord. One of the big challenges in pinpointing the reason for the loss of libido is that the differential diagnosis can be challenging, especially when a woman has multiple symptoms at the same time.

Why do I feel detached?

You may be scared of the changes; what if your partner no longer finds you desirable after menopause? What if, like Nina, you start to feel like you never want to make love to your partner again? It may feel scary because you do not want to lose that closeness with your partner and because you love connecting with him on that intimate level.

Again, my mind tells me that I may be one of those women who do not experience vaginal dryness, the loss of desire, and of course, the unsexy feeling of a body that I no longer recognize.

Then, I sober myself up, I remind myself that I very well may be, this does not sound like a 'mind over matter' problem. I know from my own experiences with hormone fluctuations that it is near impossible to 'mind-over-matter' your way out of hormonal chaos in your body. Think of this example, our hunger and satiety levels are largely controlled by the hormones Insulin and Ghrelin, it is nearly impossible to override a craving that stems from a physiological trigger such as hormones. It is the same with sex hormones, you really stand no chance against them by fighting them, so you have to learn to make them work for you.

How to rekindle intimacy?

1. **Discover New Dimensions of Intimacy**

With the physical and emotional shifts during menopause, intimacy can take on new forms. It's an opportune moment to explore beyond traditional notions of intimacy. Engage in activities like shared hobbies, long walks, or simply spending quality time together. These experiences can deepen emotional connections, proving that intimacy extends far beyond the physical realm.

2. **Schedule Intimate Time**

With the myriad of changes and possible stressors during menopause, setting aside dedicated time for intimacy can be beneficial. This doesn't necessarily mean scheduling sex, but rather creating opportunities for closeness and connection, such as date nights, cuddling sessions, or intimate conversations.

3. **Explore Sensual Activities**

Rekindling intimacy isn't limited to sexual intercourse. Explore other sensual activities like shared baths, massages, or simply holding hands. These activities can strengthen the physical and emotional bond between partners and can be especially comforting during a time of change.

How to communicate emotional changes to my partner without them feeling blamed?

As with most relationship matters, your first line of defence is to communicate. So, how do you communicate with your partner on this complex topic? When we are talking about intimacy, we are talking about so many aspects of ourselves; for women, we often talk about physical issues like lubrication (or the lack thereof), self-esteem (or the lack thereof), the state of the relationship and, of course, your hormone levels at any given time.

For men, it may be more physical, and the challenge may be in managing the male ego and helping the man understand that the lack of lust is not due to his inadequacies but rather about these very real changes happening to the woman. Sounds good, right? Well, we all also know it is probably easier said than done, these hormone fluctuations often lead to difficult conversations and relationship friction, so in truth, some of the lack of desire may be about the person, or the relationship conflict, and it becomes a very tricky balancing act between two people, navigating their own emotional and physical terrain and still trying to meet in a relationship space as well.

The keys to communication during this challenging time that I found, are actually really simple:

- Learn to regulate your own emotions - so that you always speak out of a place of wanting to have a successful conversation;
- Speak about your experiences, using "I statements" - ("I feel frustrated when...", "I would like to change the way we...", and refrain from placing blame;
- Here's the biggest tip I can give you, "LISTEN" - when you share your challenges with your partner, give him time to speak his mind. Even if you disagree, even if you want to set the record straight, give him time to speak, and when he is done, let him understand that you heard him. Like I did, you may find that the simple act of allowing him to be heard opens up communication between the two of you, and it can lead to a new level of connection and intimacy between you two.
- Be honest; while you can aim to speak gently and mindfully about your challenges, you also need to be honest. So, if, for example, you no longer enjoy the way he touches you, you need to be honest about that and be authentic about your reasons for that, as far as you understand. Know that it is not unusual for a woman to respond differently to touch after you go through menopause; being under-sensitive to touch is the most common response. This happens because the vagina changes and the vaginal walls, which are often only a few cell layers thick, become thinner. The vagina also becomes shorter and narrower as a result of hormonal changes which occur at menopause. All these changes mean you need to relearn touch and what is enjoyable for you.
- This all becomes easier and easier as you get to know yourself better. You can be very clear with your partner about what is going on with you. Reading a book like this, and perhaps even something specific to communication in

relationships, like the famous 'Men Are from Mars, Women Are from Venus,' can also help you in this journey.

Is there couple's therapy or counseling geared toward navigating these changes?

Suppose you, like me, have been in tricky relationship spots. In that case, you may have had relationship therapy, and I would always opt for this step if I realize that the partners hold so much resentment between them and that they have deteriorated so far in their communication styles with each other that they no longer can seem to connect in a constructive communication space. Sometimes, having an objective third party is just what you need.

If it is the lack of sex specifically that is putting strain on the relationship, you can even consider seeing a sex therapist who will be able to help you bridge any specific sexual issues that are showing up. A therapist can help you and your partner learn to talk openly and create a safe space to have these challenging conversations, making communication easier and easier as you learn to listen to each other again.

Case Study: Jessie gets her groove back

Let's look at my friend, Jessie. In her twenties and thirties, Jessie was always a pretty sexual person. She would often comment to her friends how much she enjoyed sex with her partner, who later became her husband, and she was one of those people who seemed to have no sexual hang-up. Even after having kids, she and Mike, her hubby, would still have regular date nights and weekends away to make time to connect with each other. When she turned 40, things changed; suddenly, she had no desire for sex, and when Mike touched her, she would cringe. She was as surprised as he was and tried to figure out what on earth was going on with her and why she stopped liking her husband's touch. It wasn't until she started noticing her period become irregular and a bit of weight gain that she realized that she might be in perimenopause.

When she realized she was in perimenopause, she made an appointment with a sex therapist, and she and Mike went for a few sessions. One of the tips the therapist shared with them was for her to explore her changing body solo, using pleasure toys so that she could rediscover what worked for her and come to trust herself and her body as a sexual being again.

It took them a few months, but I'm happy to say that today, Jessie and Mike have a renewed spark between them; the intimacy between them has grown to new depths, and they have a happy and healthy sex life, even though she has been through menopause and is now post-menopausal.

FAMILY AND FRIENDS

Nothing can prepare you for the effects of menopause on your interpersonal relationships. You may have read extensively on the effects that menopause will have on your body and mind, but what does it do to the status and strength of your emotional and spiritual network? Have you considered the work and coping mechanisms you will need to put in place in order for your relationships to survive - and, better yet, thrive during menopause?

There are natural consequences to every relationship, such as the romantic connection you have with your partner, as discussed above, which really seems quite obvious since we are talking about something so personal and so deeply rooted in feminine energy, but there are far more things to consider.

You have a multitude of relationships to bring into the balance of your menopause strategy - done right, these relationships can help you make it through this transition and even celebrate the changes that come with it. Done poorly, or worse, if you ignore the needs around relationships during menopause, you may lose the connections and destroy the relationships (or cause unnecessary conflict that you simply do not need during this time).

Can menopause affect my relationship with my children?

For many women, menopause is a shift not only from one physical experience to another, but it is a shift in identity and relationships. This is something that all women experience, but especially those that are mothers.

Many women are also becoming mothers later in life which means that they are raising young children while undergoing perimenopause and menopause. The effects of menopause, such as low mood, exhaustion brought on by sleep deprivation, anxiety, and even just a general sense of irritability, are incredibly overwhelming to experience - least of all when you have small minds and hearts to nurture.

The experience is so intense that many mothers have admitted feeling guilty about snapping at their children or simply being too tired to help them with homework or play. It has left many mothers with the distinct feeling of not coping with motherhood and very little satisfaction or enjoyment of family life.

I found some insight on this when speaking to a holistic healer when she explained that our hormones have a purpose in every stage of our lives. The hormonal shift that makes us want to draw away and put a bit of physical distance between us and our children is actually a support mechanism for mothers to start letting go as their children grow into teenagers and adults - stages when your children actually need more independence. If you keep this in mind when you think of your relationship with your children, it helps you realize that there is a *need* for change and growth, and that menopause actually facilitates this process.

So yes, menopause affects your relationship with your children, and as with any transition, it can be a difficult and emotional time - but it is also a necessary gift that allows you to become stronger in your relationship with yourself as well as your children. It is mother nature's way of saying that you can start giving back to yourself again and not solely give to your children as you have before.

Communication and openness within yourself and from your children for a need to adapt and change, as well as a sense of grace and kindness, can help you manage the way menopause affects your relationship with your children and can - dare I say it - be a blessing in disguise.

Supporting and Being Supported

The number one takeaway that comes out again and again whenever I talk with women about menopause is the need for support. Not only the act of receiving support but also the act of offering support and still being present for others while being allowed to experience menopause authentically, without feeling the need to place yourself at a disadvantage in order to make it through. This means both being vocal and clear about your support needs as well as managing and communicating your boundaries as a crutch to others.

So what does support during menopause look like? For some, it could be the simple act of a partner who can help you see the lighter side of things and, without being trivial or dismissive of the experience, can help you laugh about it all. After all, hot flashes and sweats at the wrong moment can be funny - if you choose to see the light side of it. A giggle and a supportive squeeze on the hand (because heaven forbid someone tries to hug you in the middle of a sweat-fueled heatwave) can be just the encouragement you need to keep going.

Support can also be in camaraderie and teamwork. Lifestyle and diet changes that help you better cope with menopause are so much easier to incorporate if you have a partner who will make those changes along with you.

No matter what support works best for you, this will always be true: honesty in the experience is crucial.

Addressing Awkwardness

Speaking of honesty in the experience, let's talk about when things get awkward. First let's be honest right here: menopause can be embarrassing. Not every woman feels comfortable with announcing things about her own body, let alone things that have traditionally been labeled as taboo or private.

Think about walking up to a stranger and announcing that you are on your period. Weird right? Well, no wonder then that women feel uncomfortable about addressing the fact that their hormones are waging an onslaught on their bodies, making them endure all the physical repercussions of the experience - without any room to advocate for their personal and private needs. It's time to change the narrative.

When menopause makes things awkward, address it head-on - acknowledge that it is happening, add a funny remark if you choose to lighten the situation at an appropriate time, ask for the support you need at the moment (be specific), and then move on with what you were doing. Remember, the people who matter don't mind and the people who mind don't matter.

Strengthening Bonds - how to nurture relationships and ensure they remain strong during menopause?

It remains important no matter what stage of your life you are in to nurture and strengthen your relationships with family, friends, colleagues, and even yourself. During menopause, this can feel like a tremendous undertaking, and you might not know where to start. The simplest advice is to reach out, no matter how alien it may feel at first.

Let your friends and family know that you want to engage and invest in the relationship and that while menopause can be hard to get through - it's easier when you have company and an understanding support system. Communicate how important they are to you and let them know what you are going through and how they can help.

More than anything else, be patient and kind to yourself and ask for patience and grace from those around you. Remember, building relationships on the good days means there will be relationships to fall back on when the bad days strike. Let your people know that this is what you are trying to do, and allow them to show up for you when you feel overwhelmed.

SOCIAL CIRCLES AND WORKPLACES

Since we're talking about relationships, let's take a look at the practical side of maintaining those relationships during menopause. What does it look like and what should you keep in mind when you socialize? How do you manage menopause in the workplace and maintain good standing with your inter-office relationships? Are there ways in which you can make your workplace more menopause friendly?

The best way to approach these scenarios is to be as armed with information as you can be. This will help you better communicate your need for empathy and understanding and give yourself the tools and techniques you will need to navigate social situations during menopause.

Just as with friends and family, when you use honest communication and insist on an environment of trust, kindness, and grace - you will see the results in an easier and perhaps even favorable experience in your menopause journey.

Socializing During Menopause

Studies have shown that socialization during menopause can have a positive effect not only on the general experience of menopause, but on your overall health during menopause too. In fact, it has been proven that having a social network for support during this transition reduces stress levels and improves your mental health. More than this, the research has shown that social networks have ensured that women feel more positive about menopause and that they are less likely to fall into bouts of depression.

So if socializing during menopause is so important and has wide range of benefits, then clearly, knowing how to socialize is crucial to your menopause journey. Then the question really here is how do we do that?

The first thing we need to do is to make it easy for ourselves. Do what you can to preemptively reduce barriers, including everything from incontinence underwear to a wardrobe update that favors your menopause needs. Don't just fall back on socializing like you used to. Find new ways to express yourself and connect through something you're passionate about. Try a new hobby, club, or class to get things going based on what YOU would love to do.

Throw away the rulebook! If going *out* is overwhelming, then stay *in* and invite friends over to mingle with you. Keep it low-key and low-pressure: stipulate both a start and end time and order in instead of cooking to ease the stress of hosting. You could even take things online to fill the gaps between in-person socialization -

whatever you do, remember to take it slow and release yourself from expectations.

Menopause in the Office: Navigate Relationships and Performance Amidst the Change

Navigating socialization in the workplace is a common concern for many women, especially when they feel physically overwhelmed. Maintaining relationships with your colleagues and co-workers can be tricky when you are in the midst of menopause. So what should you expect and what should you do to make the most of it?

One of the fundamental things to remember about menopause in the workplace is that women often report a significant increase in difficulty with regard to managing symptoms and interpersonal relationships. This is in large part due to the feelings of fear and embarrassment that are associated with disclosure, often creating concern about being stigmatized for being menopausal.

Many women actually report menopause as a leading consideration for wanting to leave the workplace, which is particularly alarming considering that menopausal women are the fastest-growing workforce demographic. [1] So, how do you go about that? The most important strategy is based on awareness, and if your workplace does not have a dynamic and up-to-date policy around menopause, then perhaps now is the time to initiate one.

Menopause symptoms, in particular those that affect mood, confidence, memory, and concentration - can have a devastating effect on your work and productivity. The simple act of allowing two caveats, flexible working and the ability to control the temperature in your office, can have a drastically positive effect on menopausal women in the workplace. Since the worldwide shift to hybrid or remote working, many women have found it easier to advocate for their needs and benefit from the support these environments offer them.

To that point, I recall a few incidents with a co-worker when I was a young manager. The older lady who was working for me was always complaining about the temperature in the office, and no solution seemed to help. One moment she was complaining that it was too hot and the next she was complaining about the aircon being on. I could never understand her seemingly irrational and inconsistent behavior, but today I realize she was probably suffering from flushes and the emotional turmoil of menopause, but I never had the comfort to speak openly about this subject, which was even more of a taboo topic 20 years ago.

Most importantly, prepare yourself for the effects that menopause can have on your relationships at work and decide on strategies to manage it. Opening up to your co-workers about your experience can be hugely beneficial to you and should be done with care. Be honest, explain your symptoms, and put them at ease if they have questions they would like to ask. Doing so can create an environment of support and understanding that will transform your journey.

Building Understanding and Empathy

As mentioned, for many women, a key factor in their menopause journey is the level of support they receive. When we are offered understanding and empathy, it makes the ordeal so much easier to undergo. It makes things more bearable and creates a network of love and kindness that eases the transition immensely.

In order to build this standard of understanding and empathy, you will need three main things: a proactive approach to your workplace policies, an ability to communicate and advocate for your changing needs, and a network of human beings that are willing to take on the mantle of grace and compassion on your behalf. Talk to your people and let them know what you're going through. Insist on education around the topic, an inclusive workplace culture, and formal support groups in order to make the journey better for yourself.

Let's remember of course that the social implications and support systems we have discussed here are really only one facet of your journey. It plays a significant role, but so do the healing strategies you implement to allow yourself the room and resources to make it through.

The extremely personal exercise of dealing with the physical, emotional, mental, and spiritual changes that are taking place in your life during menopause is something that womankind has been working on for centuries. For many, the practice of holistic healing and traditional medicine is the most successful and accessible option. Take what you have learned from this chapter about your relationships and apply it to your entire life - soon, you will realize that you need every available tool in your belt, which includes understanding what natural healing can do for you.

5
NATURE'S NURTURING - HOLISTIC HEALING

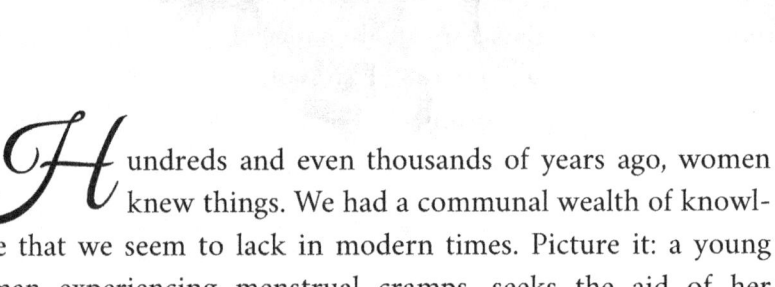

Hundreds and even thousands of years ago, women knew things. We had a communal wealth of knowledge that we seem to lack in modern times. Picture it: a young woman experiencing menstrual cramps, seeks the aid of her community healer. She is given a herbal remedy, a plant we now know as willow bark, and told to rest. Dial forward a few hundred years, and we see a Grecian woman using this same plant to ease the pain of childbirth and treat fevers. Then, in 1897, Felix Hoffmann, a Bayer chemist, synthesized aspirin - derived from the traditional knowledge of these ancient healers. It is a fact that modern medicine is derived from these natural and unassuming remedies, which is why so many women are turning back to their roots - sometimes literally.

WHAT IS HOLISTIC HEALING?

Let's take a look at what holistic healing is. At its core, holistic healing is an alternative approach to health and wellness. Alternate to what you might ask? Well, to modern (Western) medicine. The thing is, holistic healing used to be the standard, not the deviation. So, what makes it so controversial?

Holistic healing is healing based on nature (meaning that you will often come across recommendations to use plant parts, seeds, roots, and so on). It ignores the rigid verticle of pharmaceutical-style care and takes a more nuanced and collaborative approach instead. Holistic healing is an approach that simultaneously addresses the physical, mental, social, emotional, and spiritual facets of the human being. It makes room for understanding around complex and evolving needs based on multiple disciplines in health, medicine, religion, culture, environments, and communities. Holistic healing transcends a black-and-white medical approach and often incorporates things that are difficult to tally and charge for. It also challenges patriarchal views of the female body and advocates for the being and their personal needs instead of what is deemed appropriate or clinically defined.

Are there natural remedies for menopause?

Yes! There are so many natural remedies that can help you during menopause. Holistic healing offers an extensive range of options in terms of treatment as well as natural remedies that can address the symptoms of menopause quite effectively. Remedies vary from herbal supplements to lifestyle changes (such as movement, massage, or even therapies).

Holistic healing also supports the whole person in terms of the change that your body, mind, and life are undergoing. Herbal remedies such as those discussed later in this chapter can give immense relief while simultaneously making your menopausal care accessible, affordable, and totally under your own control.

Lifestyle changes to consider to support holistic healing?

Holistic healing is actually a shift in lifestyle more than anything else. The changes you may want to consider adopting when you choose a holistic path include physical wellness, such as movement (not necessarily exercise) and getting enough sleep.

Nutrition also plays a vital role in holistic wellness since many of the 'solutions' or 'treatments' for ailments are based on diet and natural sources of minerals and so on - in other words what you ingest or consume. We will look at this more in Chapter 6.

Emotional wellness is also key to holistic healing - as is spiritual, social, and intellectual wellness. To this end, practices such as yoga, meditation, self-love, and removing toxins and toxic environments from your life are essential.

Are there risks associated with holistic healing? How long does it take to see results?

Done poorly, without the proper education and safety measures, holistic approaches can become dangerous. Natural medicine is still medicine and should be treated with the same respect. It is rare that you can overdose on homeopathic treatments, but the abuse of any substance or ingredient can have unwanted effects. Some results can be seen almost immediately, such as the sleepiness and calm derived from Valerian, while other approaches may take a few months for you to truly enjoy the full benefits. It all depends on the individual in question, who is, after all, the most important beneficiary of a holistic, healthy lifestyle.

What role does stress management play in holistic healing?

Stress is one of the leading causes of misalignment and distress within the body, mind, and soul. Naturally, stress management is an incredibly valuable part of holistic wellness. Striking a balance between work, life, and play is at the center of working towards better health in every regard. Chronic stress triggers an inflammatory response in the body, which in turn affects the baseline of your health - both physical and mental. It alters the immune system in a constant stream of fight or flight and reduces your body's ability to fight infection, trauma, or disease. Cortisol (the stress hormone) can lead you to feel fatigued, irritable, have brain fog, gain weight, experience insomnia, skin irritations, and more. Sound familiar? That's right - stress and menopause have similar effects on the body and need to be treated as a matter of utmost importance.

Can holistic healing address emotional and psychological aspects of menopause, such as mood swings and anxiety?

As we have discussed, holistic healing addresses the ENTIRE being, which means that the emotional and psychological aspects of menopause are part and parcel of the strategies to manage the experience and symptoms. We do not experience life in a vacuum - nor does menopause exist solely as a physical experience. It affects every aspect of your life and being, and holistic healing has the added advantage of being able to address mood swings, anxiety, confidence, sadness, social changes, and more. That is why holistic healing, in particular, is the right path for so many women - it addresses them on the full spectrum of the experience and not just physical symptoms.

Is there scientific evidence supporting the effectiveness of holistic approaches for menopause?

There is still some debate in the medical field on the efficacy of holistic approaches for menopause, though one aspect of the approach has been universally accepted: women *need* a multi-disciplinary approach to their wellness when it comes to menopause in order to "optimize the patient's macroenvironment".
[1]

There is some scientific evidence to support the treatment and easing of symptoms in menopausal women, though the degree to which these approaches work is still in need of more exploration. Realistically, menopause primarily requires a symptom-based treatment protocol, which means that holistic strategies are often as effective (if not more so when measured against other aspects such as spiritual wellness and so on) as Western medicine.

HERBAL HEROES: NATURE'S HEALING WONDERS

There are a number of different herbal medicines that can provide a positive effect during menopause, some of which will overlap with the section where we discuss nutrition. Remember, good holistic care requires a balanced and healthy diet as well as *balanced* herbal remedies. You cannot simply use herbal medicines as a catch-all; you should use them for an added boost.

Now that we know how to use herbal remedies, let's explore what they actually are. Herbal supplements or medicines are natural and often derived from plant parts. They are commonly presented in the form of capsules, teas, extracts, powders, tablets, or fresh or dried plant parts. Here are the top ten recommended herbs and supplements for menopause:

- Black cohosh (night sweats, hot flashes)
- Red clover (night sweats, hot flashes, bone loss)
- Dong quai (supports Black cohosh and Red clover, general PMS/menopause support)
- Evening primrose oil (hot flashes, bone loss)
- Maca (diminished sex drive, moodiness, vaginal dryness)
- Soy (general support, hot flashes, bone loss)
- Flax seeds (hot flashes, bone loss)
- Ginseng (immune function, heart health, energy levels, sex drive, mood)

- Valerian root (insomnia, hot flashes)
- Chasteberry (anxiety, hot flashes)

A friendly warning: just because these herbal remedies are natural does not mean they are safe to use indiscriminately. Always check in with your healthcare provider before using herbal remedies or medicines, and ensure that you use the correct amounts.

Phytoestrogens: Friend or foe?

Let's start with the basics: what are phytoestrogens? Phytoestrogens have a chemical makeup similar to the estrogen that our bodies naturally produce and they are found in plants. Plants release phytoestrogens as a means of curbing the population numbers of small animals (since estrogen lowers the chances of falling pregnant). While phytoestrogens are not quite strong enough to significantly affect humans in this way, they are quite effective as a natural supplement to ease the symptoms of low estrogen.

Good sources of phytoestrogens are flax and sesame seeds, ginseng, soy (though be careful not to choose over-processed products here), oats, legumes or beans, barley, and coffee, to name a few.

Since every woman's journey is different and estrogen levels vary, it is important to note that an overdose of phytoestrogens can be as harmful as the lack of estrogen. It is important then, to always have your estrogen levels checked *before* using phytoestrogens as a remedy.

Tea Time: Beneficial herbal brews

Many herbal supplements are best ingested in the form of a herbal tea. Some already come presented in tea form, and others you may need to brew yourself using the raw ingredient. For the crafty or the resourceful women out there, you could always use tea strainers, pre-made tea bags, or even make your own tea bags. For a no-frills approach, I would just put the ingredients directly into a stewing pot or teacup, though it may be appropriate to strain the tea before drinking in many cases.

Here are some of the most beneficial (and even some of the tastiest) herbal teas you should be making to better support your body, spirit, and mind during menopause:

- Black cohosh root (used to combat vaginal dryness or hot flashes - very effective for women experiencing early menopause)
- Ginseng (try for an increase in sexual appetite as well as overall menopausal symptom relief and even to support bone formation)
- Chasteberry tree (increases progesterone and assists with hormonal balance; also good for breast pain and hot flashes)
- Red raspberry leaf (used during perimenopause to ease menstrual symptoms, especially if you are experiencing a heavy flow)
- Red clover (boosts immunity, supports bone strength, and is sometimes used to treat high blood pressure, contains phytoestrogens)

Adaptogens: Nature's stress-busters

Before we close off the chapter on herbal medicines, we need to look at one of the most crucial parts of your holistic healing regime: adaptogens.

First, what are adaptogens? Adaptogens are known as nature's response to stress - active substances found in certain herbs and plants that can improve the way your body responds to stress. The practice has been used for centuries in Chinese and Ayurvedic medicine as a natural approach to lowering stress and anxiety and improving your overall well-being. We have access to many known adaptogens, including household favorites such as Ginseng and Turmeric. In order for us to classify a substance as an adaptogen it has to be non-toxic in normal amounts; effective throughout the entire body against stress; and support homeostasis or the return to an ideal balanced state.

Some examples of adaptogens include: Ashwagandha, Ginseng, Turmeric, Tulsi (Holy Basil), Eleuthero, Liquorice, Goji berry, and Golden root (Rhodiola Rosea).

MINDFUL METHODS

Many women find strength and power in dealing with their menopause journey by activating their higher self and leveraging the strongest tool in their arsenal- the mind. Not only has this been a tried-and-trusted route for women for centuries now, but it engages us on our most cerebral and spiritual level, something that transcends the physical reality of the symptoms of discomfort.

For some women, menopause marks an incredibly important transition in their lives having gone through the stages from maiden to mother and now to sage. It is a transformation in themselves not only of physical discourse but of spiritual and mental evolution as well. It is a matter of pride and satisfaction that their 'wise old years' are upon them and they can revel in the beauty and glory that comes with being a woman in her spiritual prime. In fact, it is widely believed that this is the era of womanhood that is most rewarding and, in fact, necessary for familial and societal structures. These women have their places firmly secured within the tapestry of their social network and engage on an ethereal plane with those around them.

Stepping away for a moment from the esoteric high-level ideals, all of which are appropriate and applicable to the feminine journey, let us explore the practical ways in which you can use mindful methods to heal during menopause.

Meditation and Mindfulness

Meditation is the art of focused concentration in which you return to a moment or matter repeatedly, returning over and over again to address stress and dissipate it - regardless of whether this is a positive or negative experience. It emphasizes the need for concentration and clarity in order to ease the mind. Mindfulness, an extension of meditation, is the act of focusing on being totally and intensely aware of what you are sensing and feeling at any given moment, free from the confines of judgment or interpretation. Mindfulness meditation allows us to experience a state of awareness and acceptance of the physical realm without succumbing to it in the moment.

Studies have shown that women who have a higher mindfulness score (as recorded in a study done at Mayo Clinic[2]) experience fewer symptoms of menopause. Other research[3] shows us that mindfulness creates several positive psychological effects, including wellness and behavioral regulation.

In my experience, the simple act of using mindfulness and meditation in your day-to-day life can have a dramatic impact on your experience of menopause. You could even start today with some simple mindful exercises, such as word repetition and paced breathing exercises, or even by incorporating a mindfulness app that will prompt you through the experience.

My favorite apps to recommend are:

- Balance
- Calm

- Headspace
- Insight Timer
- Breethe
- Portal

Yoga's Yin and Yang: Best poses for menopause

Another wonderful mindful practice that women turn to for relief and healing during menopause is that of yoga. Yoga has been the go-to for restoration and rejuvenation for centuries and allows you to unlock a physical level of healing as well as a mental and spiritual one. Many women have actively sought out yoga, especially for the benefits it poses for stress and pain relief, two of the major physical factors in hormonal changes.

Here are some of the best poses you can incorporate into your yoga regime for better support and restoration in your menopause journey.

For stress relief, digestive aid, and depression:

- Shoulderstand
- Marichyasana A
- Head-to-knee Forward Bend

For hot flashes:

- Supta Baddha Konasana (Reclining Bound Angle Pose)
- Adho Mukha Svanasana (Downward-Facing Dog)
- Supta Virasana (Reclining Hero Pose)
- Setu Bandha Sarvangasana (Bridge Pose)
- Prasarita Padottanasana (Wide-Legged Forward Bend)

Incorporating yoga into your daily routine is a great way to deal with the symptoms of menopause, but it also offers you so much more in terms of wellness for physical, mental, and spiritual health and wealth.

Breath Work and Its Benefits

Breath work is another tool that combats both the physical and the mental or cognitive symptoms of menopause. Used correctly, it can offer you immense symptomatic relief and increased focus to alleviate the fogginess that comes with this stage of your journey. Using "in-breaths" (breathing in through your nose) ensures a higher rate of oxygen intake and therefore mental clarity. Focused deep breathing techniques will help you think clearer and offer you a boost of mental energy just when you need it most.

Deep breathing is also a relaxation technique that can provide you with much-needed support during menopause - it can be quite stressful, after all! Breathwork is a biological, cognitive, and emotional support that can release the negative burden of menopause and replace it with deep focus, relaxation, feelings of peacefulness, and, for bonus points, a slower heart rate (this helps with overall physical rejuvenation, too).

THERAPEUTIC TOUCH

Therapeutic touch has offered many women deep and healing support during some of the most traumatic and difficult times in their lives. It has been shown to improve sleep and quality of life and reduce the symptoms of menopause as well.

I remember talking to Anya, a good friend of mine from work, and we found ourselves lamenting about the difficult week we had just had and musing about the ways in which we wanted to unwind and destress. Anya pointed out that she had managed her stress levels far better than usual, and I realized she was right. This was quite a milestone for her, too, since she had been dealing with menopause for the greater part of a year at this point. When I quizzed her about the magic recipe, she revealed to me that she had been going for weekly treatments, alternating massage, and acupuncture and that while the week had been trying, she knew that she would feel more like herself again after her appointment.

Years later, when I was in the thick of dealing with menopause, I remembered this moment, and I immediately booked myself in for a reflexology massage. Naturally, I still needed to do a lot of research and self-education before I fully understood how best to use therapeutic touch and also why it works, but I felt the benefit of having that insider secret ready to go, not to mention the benefits of the massage on my physical, mental, emotional, and spiritual well being. From that day on, I knew I had to delve a little deeper.

Therapeutic touch, especially when coupled with music therapy can be incredibly rewarding and cathartic. Considering that, on average, 50% of women report having issues with sleep during menopause (reports tally 40% to 60%[4]), this is an important and useful find. Again, we are seeing that complementary and alternative medicine (CAM) offers women new avenues for responding to their needs during menopause.

Therapeutic touch includes any practice that uses studied systems of touch or healing to address an individual's physiological, cognitive, and spiritual wellness. Examples include (but are not limited to) acupuncture, massage, reflexology, biofeedback, hypnosis, aromatherapy, and more. Let's discuss the three primary touch-based therapies below.

Acupuncture Explained

Acupuncture is an ancient practice that falls under traditional Chinese medical techniques. An acupuncturist is a trained, professional practitioner who uses thin needles inserted into the skin at specific points on the body (known as acupuncture points and based on the flow of qi - our vital energy - running through the body). Once the needles are placed in position, they remain there for approximately 20 minutes to stimulate and invigorate the energy. During this process, the body also releases endorphins (otherwise known as mother nature's painkiller).

While it is important to note that acupuncture in itself cannot control pain, it does have the ability to increase the blood flow and the body's natural response to alleviate the symptoms associated with both pain and menopause in general. This means that it can, as a result of the process, offer effective pain relief.

Acupuncture can target these symptoms specifically:

- Hot flashes
- Night sweats
- Fatigue
- Insomnia
- Mood swings
- Headaches
- Anxiety
- Palpitations
- Depression
- Pain

Acupuncture addresses these and a host of more nuanced symptoms that occur due to the symptoms above.

Massage Magic

There are a number of massage techniques that are firm favorites when it comes to releasing tension and discomfort during menopause. I loved getting massages when I was having a particularly difficult week - it felt like I was rewarding myself to make it through and giving myself an extra dose of coping for the next stretch (or at least until my next massage!). To some women, massage feels overly indulgent, but as someone who has suffered for years with my menstrual symptoms, when it came to menopause, I thought it was finally time to give myself a bit more nurturing and care - and it paid off.

The top massage types recommended for menopause include:

Swedish massage - which focuses on increased circulation and relaxation. The therapist will often use oils and lotions to facilitate the gliding motions required.

Shiatsu - focuses energy and blood flow. This treatment is used to release toxins and deep-seated tensions.

Myofascial release - addresses poor posture, emotional stress, and physical injury or illness. It focuses on the connective tissue layer surrounding the muscles, bones, and joints.

Reflexology's Rationale

Reflexology is another amazing alternative therapy that benefits women going through menopause. Not only is it based on the scientific method, but it wholesomely incorporates the higher self into the treatment as well. Reflexologists are commonly therapists or will, at the very least, be there to listen and advise you during your session. It can be hugely releasing and empowering while at the same time giving physical relief from discomfort. Importantly, reflexology is a combination treatment that addresses physical, mental, emotional, and spiritual wellness.

Reflexology can regulate the peripheral nervous system by stimulating specific reflex points, namely the thymus, hypothalamus, and pituitary gland. As a therapy during menopause, it can offer relief from stress and tension as well as offer a cleansing of the body and emotions to bring balance back to your hormonal levels.

Try reflexology if you want to tackle anxiety, depression, night sweats, and hot flashes head-on.

Now that we have explored the gentle, holistic, and natural approaches, let's pivot slightly towards a more aggressive intervention-type strategy: Hormone Replacement Therapy. I am sure you may be very curious about it.

UNDERSTAND HRT: EXPLORE ITS RISKS AND BENEFITS

HRT stands for Hormone Replacement Therapy. HRT is medication containing female hormones that are used to replace the estrogen in your body that you stop producing during menopause.

HRT has proven beneficial in instances of menopause based on the decrease in the intensity of symptoms. It has also been proved to reduce instances of bone loss and lower the risk of fractures in postmenopausal women.

While there are a host of benefits to HRT, we must also be aware of the indicated risks. Depending on the type of hormone therapy, as well as the dose and duration of use, there may be serious negative side effects on your overall health. You may be more at risk of stroke, heart disease, blood clots, and even breast cancer if you use hormone replacement therapy that has not been perfectly calibrated to your body.

It is advised when thinking about HRT that you consult with your healthcare professional about the type of product and delivery method that would be best for you. You should also try to minimize the amount of medication you take, follow through with regular follow-up care, and make overall healthy life choices.

How and why was HRT developed?

Let's explore where HRT comes from. Well, as is the usual course of medical discovery and advancement [5], it came from a more realistic perspective on menopause that was provided by research on the endocrine system during which the ovarian hormones were isolated. The belief that menopause symptoms were actually symptoms of madness was replaced by a theory that "a woman's lost femininity" could be restored through hormone treatments.

One of the first treatments in this field, Ovariin, was created using pulverized cow ovaries blended with a flavored powder. Another subsequent treatment called Emminen was created using the urine of pregnant women; this was later replaced with a more cost-effective drug called Premarin, which utilized the urine of pregnant mares. The treatment gained popularity in the 1960s and was later found to help reduce a woman's risk for breast cancer, heart attack, and stroke. These findings were, however, later refuted as over-enthusiastic and were balanced out with the research on the long-term effects and risks of HRT.

HRT Variations and Options

Today there are quite a few more options available. HRT is provided in two main types, namely combined HRT (estrogen and progestogen) and estrogen-only HRT. The former is used for women who still have their wombs and the latter for those who have had a hysterectomy. There are a number of types of HRT including the patch, the implant, tablets, gels, or sprays. BHRT, or Bioidentical Hormone Replacement Therapy (meaning identical to human biology), is also an option available today. This treatment is man-made, and as it is bioidentical, in other words chemically identical to the ones that are made by your body, it is easily absorbable.

Beyond the method of administration, it's important to consider individual factors such as age, health history, and specific symptoms when choosing the right type of HRT. Additionally, the duration of HRT use is a critical aspect, typically tailored based on personal health risks and benefits. Regular consultation with healthcare professionals is essential for monitoring and adjusting treatment as needed. This approach ensures that each woman receives personalized care, maximizing the benefits of HRT while minimizing potential risks. Understanding these diverse options and considerations empowers women to make informed decisions about their hormonal health during menopause

Western Medicine

Unlike modern medical rhetoric, holistic healing holds a place for Western medicine - that is to say, while holistic healing shows a preference for herbal and holistic remedies and treatment, it does not ignore nor seek to replace valuable treatment that Western medicine can offer.

A good example is how holistic healers look at Western medicine for menopause. Western medicine offers access to HRT (Hormone Replacement Therapy) as a treatment option - and you could take a holistic approach to ensure that you are treating the very specific situation of each patient in terms of her hormone levels and other contributing medical conditions. In fact, there was even a study done on the use of a combined approach in which "the results showed that when compared with patients using only HRT, the total clinical response rate is greater in patients using HRT combined with one of these 12 oral Chinese patent medicines [6]."

To this end, we look at the various options available for treating menopause based in Western medicine:

- Hormone Replacement Therapy or MHT (Menopausal Hormone Therapy)
- Vaginal estrogen

- Low-dose antidepressants - for decreasing menopausal hot flashes
- Gabapentin (Gralise, Horizant, Neurontin) - used to treat seizures but useful to combat nighttime hot flashes
- Clonidine (Catapres, Kapvay) - used to treat high blood pressure but can offer relief from hot flashes
- Fezolinetant (Veozah) - hormone free, works by blocking the neural pathway that regulates body temperature
- Osteoporosis medication to alleviate the symptoms of bone loss and degeneration

Overall, Western medicine offers scientific and chemical treatment options that natural options do not, and Western options are far more intensive in their results. In contrast, natural options are more mild in effect.

There are so many incredible ways in which we can better address the symptoms and overall experience of menopause, specifically in the way we approach healing. A holistic approach allows us the freedom and nuance of seeing ourselves as whole beings, varied and with a myriad of balancing needs, that deserve to be treated as more than a walking list of symptoms.

Women have for generations looked to their elders or ancestral guides for insight on menopause and though we may seem to have lost a great deal of this culture, we still benefit from holistic healing in a large way. Natural remedies, physical therapy, and really all of the techniques and tools we have listed in this chapter are making a resurgence that I personally am very happy to see. Every woman should know about which teas to drink or which yoga positions to use to better support her through her menopause journey. Thankfully, these methods are becoming ever more popular and we can start seeing the benefits of living as whole beings through menopause.

Naturally, there is more to this than simply holistic remedies. As I have discussed previously, the right approach to menopause requires balance, specifically the balance of supplements and nutrition. Good nourishment and a healthy diet can make a world of difference and are required for a strong menopause strategy.

∼

6
NOURISH AND FLOURISH THROUGH MENOPAUSE

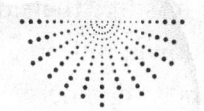

You are what you eat; we've all heard that, and I have always been a relatively healthy eater, better than my peers anyway, but I could (and did) always count on my body bouncing back quickly from an indulgent weekend of decadent food and alcohol-fueled festivities. That was until I crashed into perimenopause. I say 'crashed' because, for me, it did not happen gently; as I entered my 40th year on earth, my body just changed almost overnight. I literally have pictures of myself 7 days apart, before my mom's 60th birthday weekend and after that, it is like my body had not recovered from that one long weekend of indulgence.

It took me a year of self-loathing about my lack of discipline to get back in shape and good health, until I realized that my body had geared down into perimenopause, at that exact same time, (one month after I entered my forties), and the perfect storm occurred, leaving me feeling fat, depleted, and sad.

The great news is that I reversed most of that damage, and today, I am happy, healthy, and in the best shape of my life.

Let's look at how you can use food as medicine to help you master menopause in the most powerful way.

METABOLISM SHIFT: UNDERSTAND THE SLOWDOWN

Here's the thing: when you hit perimenopause, it's like everything slows down, the entire show goes into slo-mo. This was my experience: The best way I can describe it is like a cloud of angelic music descended on me; it is like the cloud hypnotized my entire being-ness into slowing down, movement around me, my breath, the wind, sound, light and…my energy…like the entire universe told me: *"slow down, reflect, reconsider, this is your time to reinvent yourself, you're at a crossroad and I am forcing you to make a conscious choice about what your future will look like…"*

Sounds romantic, right? Well, it was on the one hand, but on the other, not so much, because with this slowing down came a slower metabolism; it led to weight gain, which led to anxiety at first, depression later, and apathy when I reached a point of such hopelessness that I didn't really care about the weight anymore (at least on the surface level).

How can I manage weight gain during menopause through diet?

I was feeling really bad about my body, to the point that I did not find any activities enjoyable (not even a trip to a tropical island with my partner because I didn't want to have to get into a bikini). I realized I had to stop and look at how I was treating my body. I realized that, yes, I had to move more, but I also had to reconsider what I would be putting into my body in the future.

I started studying nutrition on every level and learned about the nutritional value of food as taught by modern science, and about the energetic or spiritual impact of food.

I decided to find a balance between Western medicine recommendations and my body's own intuitive knowledge. I would also incorporate Ayurvedic medicine and look at the spiritual perspective of different religions to find the true wisdom behind the reasoning for limiting (or eliminating) the intake of certain foods.

In the rest of this chapter, I will relay to you some Western nutritional recommendations, which is what you will find in most books about menopause, and I will also share (where I feel it adds value) some of the more spiritual aspects of diet that helped me.

Portion control is key

This is one thing you will not be able to get away from. As your metabolism slows down during perimenopause and menopause, your body burns less energy for fuel, and whatever is not burned is stored as fat. It is really that simple, and for this reason, it becomes very important to be mindful of your portions. Make sure you consume enough high-nutritional foods and move away from eating meals or snacks that are low in nutrition but high in energy (calories).

POWER FOODS: BOOST HORMONAL HARMONY AND ENERGY

Now, let's look at some specific foods that can fuel your body, become the medicine you need to thrive, and also help restore balance in your hormones.

Macronutrient Mastery: Carbs, proteins, fats

What are macronutrients, or 'macros'? These are the larger food groups that we, as humans, consume to fuel our bodies. Our three macronutrient groups are carbohydrates, fat, and protein, and in the long term, if you can establish a balance of these macros that work for you, you will have a much easier time managing your health and balancing your hormones. One of the easiest ways to do this, without getting into daily macro counting, is to ensure that all your meals include a combination of protein, carbs, and fat, and also always avoid skipping meals.

Each of the macros has a different purpose and a different working in your body, let's look at a simple summary of this:

- **Carbohydrates** are the primary fuel source, giving you the energy for your muscles and central nervous system to function when moving.
- **Protein** provides structure to the tissues in your body, like cell membranes, organs, muscle, hair, skin, nails, bones, tendons, ligaments, and blood plasma, and are involved in metabolic, hormonal and enzyme systems, helping your body maintain its acid-base balance.
- **Fat** is important as an energy reserve; it insulates and protects your organs and helps your body absorb and transport fat-soluble vitamins.

What role does protein play in menopause nutrition?

Protein supports muscle strength and tone, which is particularly important for us since women can lose up to 40 percent of their muscle mass by the time they have completed their journey through menopause. Our bone strength, nails, skin, and hair are all made up of protein, too - which is another good reason to ensure that we address our protein intake needs during menopause. Menopausal women have the risk of losing muscle mass and bone strength as their estrogen starts to decline. To help against this, women over 50 should have 0.45–0.55 grams of protein per pound daily, or 20–25 grams per meal. Protein should make up 10–35% of total daily calories.

You might also be interested to know that only 5g of collagen peptides a day can improve bone density in postmenopausal women; dairy protein is linked to an 8% lower hip fracture risk, while plant protein is linked to a 12% reduction.

Here are some foods you can include in your diet to ensure you get enough proteins: Eggs, meat, fish, legumes, dairy; vegan-friendly options are tofu, tempeh, lentils, chickpeas, quinoa, nuts and seeds, nutritional yeast, and plant-based protein powders.

Micronutrient Magnates: Vitamins and minerals

Let's talk about vitamins and minerals for a moment. Just now, we spoke about macros, I see this as the visible, physical component of nutrition, and while that is important and easier to manage because it is so tangible, the real difference in your diet that you can make is to start ensuring that you get all the minerals and vitamins that your body needs to thrive.

Vitamins are made by plants and animals, and therefore, they are called 'organic substances'. On the other hand, minerals are inorganic elements, as they come from soil and water; plants absorb them, or animals eat them. For some of these, your body needs large amounts (like calcium to support growth and long-term health) and other minerals like chromium, copper, iodine, iron, selenium, and zinc; you only need little bits of them. Hence, they are called trace minerals.

There are two categories of minerals and vitamins: fat soluble and water soluble ones. The fat-soluble vitamins are A, D, E, and K, they dissolve in fat and are stored in your body.

The water-soluble vitamins are C and B-complex vitamins (vitamins B6, B12, niacin, riboflavin, and folate), which dissolve in water, so your body can't store these vitamins. This means that any B or C vitamins that aren't used by your body will travel through your bloodstream and be expelled through your urine. This, of course, means that you need to consume these every day to fuel your body.

Foods that help with mood swings and emotional well-being

For me, everything started changing when I redefined the purpose of food in my life. I went from seeing food as entertainment, a soothing mechanism, and a regular habit, and I started looking at food as medicine. One of the most significant benefits of this repositioning in my mind is that I managed to use food to improve my mood and my emotional well-being.

Here are the specific foods I recommend to make you feel your best every day:

- **Omega-3 Fatty Acids:** You can get this from flax seeds, chia seeds, and hemp seeds or in fatty fish (mackerel, salmon), and it helps reduce low moods.
- **Fruits and Vegetables:** Fruits and vegetables are good for you on so many levels, and eating more of these natural gifts from planet earth is a certain way to improve your overall health. Eating lots of fruits and veggies can reduce your hot flashes by up to 19% and makes you feel happier. Dark berries and grape seed extract also improves mood and sleep for some of us.
- **Phytoestrogens:** Some of the compounds that can be found in foods like soybeans, chickpeas, peanuts, flax seeds, barley, berries and tea - it increases mood and emotional well-being.

FOODS TO FORSAKE

Inflammatory Culprits

As your estrogen decreases, so inflammation in your body increases. Most of us know that prolonged systemic inflammation can lead to all kinds of nasties like artery, organ, and joint damage, raising your risk of chronic diseases such as heart disease, arthritis, and dementia.

While hormone therapy may reportedly help with inflammation, you can do a lot yourself by following an anti-inflammatory diet, exercising, and implementing some lifestyle changes.

When you focus on consuming fruits, vegetables, and foods rich in unsaturated fats like avocado, fatty fish, nuts, and olive, and when you limit your intake of inflammatory-contributing foods such as ultra-processed refined carbs, sugary beverages, processed meats, and fried foods; you will start noticing how your body responds with more energy and fewer adverse symptoms. If you want to look at an off-the-shelf, tried, and tested diet, the Mediterranean and MIND diets are known for their anti-inflammatory properties. These types of diets also support bone health during menopause and towards the end of this chapter, I will share with you a bonus hormone balancing diet based on the popular Meditiranean diet.

Sugar and Menopause

Your reproductive hormones protect you against the harmful effects of sugar in your youth, but as you age and these hormones decrease in your body, so does the protection these hormones give you.

What does this mean? It means that as we get older, we need to look more closely at how much sugar we are consuming and also keep in mind that decreasing estrogen and progesterone levels can result in insulin resistance, causing higher blood sugar levels and increasing your risk for type 2 diabetes, heart disease, and some cancers, as well as causing weight gain and fatigue.

Need another reason to quit sugar? Not only can excessive sugar intake worsen menopausal symptoms, but hormone replacement therapy (HRT) may also become less effective in the management of menopausal symptoms if you have insulin resistance.

What are the pros of reducing sugar intake? Lower risk of heart disease, diabetes, and certain types of cancers, easier weight management, better overall diet, and fewer blood sugar fluctuations.

The only cons of reducing sugar include the challenge of adjusting to the taste and ubiquity of sugar in various foods. So, how can you begin to reduce your sugar intake? The best way is to start cooking at home, read the labels, get informed about nutrition, choose real foods over processed ones, and incorporate natural sugars from fruits. Remember, too, that you have plenty of options! Maple syrup, agave, honey are much healthier (and tastier in my opinion) alternatives.

Alcohol and Caffeine's Ambiguity

Alcohol and caffeine are the building blocks of a busy woman's diet during your working years. Caffeine to get you going on those super demanding days, and alcohol to help you unwind after a long day.

The trouble is that it has been found that alcohol consumption can increase menopause symptoms like hot flashes, sleep disruption, and depression, and if you are having more than 2 drinks per day or 10 drinks per week, that is something you should look at.

Heavy drinking can also increase your risk of osteoporosis as it can cause you to lose calcium and other nutrients. It also may lead to falls and fractured bones. At the same time, caffeine can trigger hot flashes, anxiety, and keep you up as a result of its stimulant effect and the hot flashes.

While managing all of these changes, symptoms, remedies, and requirements that come with having a successful menopause may seem daunting, the reward is great in the end if you persist. You take this time in your life to learn the lessons it has in store for you and cultivate a life of health, vitality, and deep-seated purpose and meaning... the promised land will be yours to enjoy...

Now that you have a good understanding of what fods will benefit you as you move through your menopause journey, I will share with you the Meditiranean Menopause Diet that I have formulated, with female hormone balancing in mind.

MENOMEDITERRANEAN HARMONY: A CULINARY GUIDE TO MENOPAUSE MASTERY

INTRODUCTION: MENOPAUSE MEDITERRANEAN DIET

As you have seen from the book, a holistic approach is the most successful way to navigate the transformative journey of menopause, and the importance of nutrition cannot be overstated. Because I understand just how important what you eat is in managing your menopause successfully, I have created a specialized diet plan called the Menopause Mediterranean Diet.

Drawing inspiration from the renowned Mediterranean diet, celebrated for its heart-healthy benefits, I infused it with a nuanced understanding of menopausal hormonal shifts and the therapeutic potential of herbs and adaptogens. As with all meal plans, this is not a one-size-fits-all solution but a thoughtful exploration into crafting a diet that aligns with the unique needs of women during this significant life stage.

I have seamlessly integrated phytoestrogen-rich foods, adaptogenic herbs, and herbal teas known for their menopause-supportive properties into the traditional Mediterranean Diet with the aim to alleviate symptoms and foster a holistic sense of well-being, acknowledging that menopause is a multifaceted experience.

It's important to remember that this diet is not a rigid prescription but a flexible guide, designed to be adapted to each individual's needs. Aim to select organic choices whenever possible, and for meat, prioritize the highest quality options, such as wild-caught and free-range, to ensure the most natural and beneficial choices.

This diet can be easily adapted for those on a plant-based diet, using alternatives like soy, tofu, and beans. This plant-based adaptation can be particularly beneficial, avoiding potential artificial hormones found in animal products.

Before starting this diet, it's recommended to consult with healthcare professionals to tailor dietary choices to individual health needs and preferences. The goal is to create a lifestyle that supports you through menopause, and even partial adherence to this plan can make a significant positive impact on your body.

WEEKLY MEDITERRANEAN MENOPAUSE DIET WITH ADAPTOGENS:

DAY 1:

Breakfast: Greek yogurt parfait with fresh berries, honey, and a sprinkle of flaxseeds. Add a pinch of Tulsi (Holy Basil) to the honey for an herbal twist.

Lunch: Quinoa salad with chickpeas, cherry tomatoes, cucumbers, feta cheese, and a lemon vinaigrette. Infuse the vinaigrette with a bit of Tulsi.

Herbal Tea Snack: Enjoy a cup of Red Raspberry Leaf tea with a slice of licorice root for sweetness.

Dinner: Grilled salmon with roasted vegetables (zucchini, bell peppers, and cherry tomatoes) and a side of barley. Use a marinade with ginseng and a touch of Goji berry for added flavor.

Snack: Handful of almonds with a few Goji berries.

DAY 2:

Breakfast: Mediterranean-style omelet with spinach, tomatoes, olives, and feta cheese. Sprinkle turmeric into the egg mixture for added color and health benefits.

Lunch: Whole grain wrap with hummus, mixed greens, and grilled chicken. Add a pinch of turmeric to the hummus for extra flavor.

Herbal Tea Snack: Herbal tea made from Chasteberry.

Dinner: Pasta with a tomato-based sauce, shrimp, and a variety of vegetables. Sprinkle with parsley and turmeric for added taste and color.

Snack: Fresh fruit (e.g., apple slices with almond butter).

DAY 3:

Breakfast: Whole grain toast with avocado and smoked salmon. Add a pinch of ashwagandha to the avocado for an earthy flavor.

Lunch: Lentil soup with a side of Greek salad (tomatoes, cucumbers, olives, and feta). Infuse the soup with Eleuthero for adaptogenic benefits.

Herbal Tea Snack: Enjoy a cup of Red Clover tea with a hint of licorice root.

Dinner: Baked cod with quinoa and steamed broccoli. Season the cod with a turmeric-infused olive oil dressing.

Snack: Yogurt with a drizzle of honey.

DAY 4:

Breakfast: Smoothie with soy milk, frozen berries, a banana, and a tablespoon of chia seeds. Add a pinch of turmeric to the smoothie for an anti-inflammatory kick.

Lunch: Spinach and chickpea salad with cherry tomatoes, red onion, and a balsamic vinaigrette. Infuse the vinaigrette with a bit of Eleuthero.

Herbal Tea Snack: Enjoy a cup of Ginseng tea with a slice of licorice root.

Dinner: Stir-fried tofu with mixed vegetables (broccoli, bell peppers, and snap peas) over brown rice. Add turmeric to the stir-fry sauce.

Snack: Mixed nuts and dried fruit.

DAY 5:

Breakfast: Overnight oats made with oats, almond milk, and chia seeds and topped with fresh fruit. Mix ashwagandha into the oats for added adaptogenic benefits.

Lunch: Quinoa-stuffed bell peppers with black beans, corn, and tomatoes. Season the stuffing with turmeric and a bit of Eleuthero.

Herbal Tea Snack: Enjoy a cup of Black Cohosh tea with a hint of licorice root.

Dinner: Grilled mackerel with a side of asparagus and quinoa. Use a marinade with ginseng and a touch of Goji berry for added flavor.

Snack: Greek yogurt with a handful of walnuts and a few Goji berries.

DAY 6:

Breakfast: Scrambled eggs with sautéed mushrooms, tomatoes, and spinach. Add a pinch of ashwagandha to the eggs for an earthy flavor.

Lunch: Falafel salad with mixed greens, cucumber, tomato, and tahini dressing. Incorporate golden root (Rhodiola Rosea) into the tahini for adaptogenic properties.

Herbal Tea Snack: Enjoy a cup of Red Clover tea with a slice of licorice root.

Dinner: Chicken souvlaki skewers with roasted vegetables and a side of whole grain couscous. Marinate the chicken with turmeric and lemon.

Snack: Fresh fruit (e.g., orange slices).

DAY 7:

Breakfast: Whole grain pancakes with fresh berries and a dollop of Greek yogurt. Add turmeric to the pancake batter.

Lunch: Mediterranean-style bowl with grilled shrimp, quinoa, cherry tomatoes, olives, and feta. Sprinkle turmeric on the shrimp.

Herbal Tea Snack: Enjoy a cup of Ginseng tea with a slice of licorice root.

Dinner: Whole wheat spaghetti with tomato and vegetable sauce, topped with grilled chicken. Add turmeric to the sauce for flavor.

Snack: Hummus with carrot and cucumber sticks, sprinkled with a few Goji berries.

This is simply a sample menu; feel free to adapt and substitute it with your favorites, while keeping in mind that variety is important to get the full benefits of all the items we are suggesting.

Notes:

Turmeric Integration: Turmeric can be added to various dishes, providing both flavor and potential health benefits.

Ginseng: Consider adding ginseng to herbal teas or soups, as mentioned in your chapter.

Herbal Teas: Choose teas based on personal preference, and consider rotating them throughout the week.

Phytoestrogens: Incorporate soy-based products, flaxseeds, and sesame seeds into meals or snacks.

Adaptogens: Rotate adaptogens like ashwagandha, Eleuthero, Tulsi, Licorice, Goji berry, and Golden root (Rhodiola Rosea) to ensure variety and balance.

Hydration: Continue to drink plenty of water throughout the day.

SHOPPING LIST*

*Buy organic, free range, and wild caught where possible

Proteins:

Fresh wild-caught salmon fillets

Free-range chicken breast

Organic tofu

Wild-caught cod fillets

Wild-caught mackerel fillets

Free-range eggs

Hummus (look for brands with natural ingredients)

Falafel mix

Whole Grains:

Quinoa

Organic barley

Whole grain wraps (look for brands with minimal additives)

Whole wheat spaghetti

Brown rice

Whole grain couscous

Whole grain pancake mix

Whole grain bread

Vegetables:

Zucchini

Bell peppers (variety of colors)

Cherry tomatoes

Cucumbers

Spinach

Avocado

Broccoli

Asparagus

Red onion

Mushrooms

Mixed greens

Fruits:

Berries (strawberries, blueberries, raspberries)

Banana

Apple

Orange

Lemon (for juice and zest)

Fruit for snacking (e.g., apple slices, orange segments)

Dairy and Dairy Alternatives: (Free range, or grass-fed where possible)

Greek yogurt

Feta cheese

Soy milk

Almond milk

Nuts and Seeds:

Almonds

Walnuts

Chia seeds

Flaxseeds

Sesame seeds

Legumes:

Chickpeas

Lentils

Black beans

Herbs and Spices:

Parsley

Cilantro

Oregano

Basil

Turmeric powder

Red chili flakes

Cumin

Paprika

Garlic powder

Oils and Condiments:

Extra virgin olive oil

Balsamic vinegar

Honey

Tahini

Hummus

Greek salad dressing

Herbal Teas and Adaptogens:

Red Raspberry Leaf tea

Chasteberry tea

Black Cohosh tea

Ginseng tea

Licorice root

Goji berries

Ashwagandha

Tulsi (Holy Basil) tea or dried leaves

Golden root (Rhodiola Rosea) capsules

∼

7
LIFE AFTER MENOPAUSE - THE PROMISED LAND

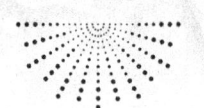

Imagine your life the way it could be: No periods. No mental gymnastics thinking about your birth control (and none of the yucky side effects). No need to worry about buying pads, or tampons, or safeguarding your underwear - just in case. For many women it also means a massive sigh of relief since they no longer have to worry about falling pregnant. For whatever reason, being post menopausal is a time to celebrate. This is YOUR TIME and you have earned your freedom.

Women have for centuries been really good at looking after others - as nurturers, as creators of life, even just as a shoulder to cry on when someone needs empathy and understanding. Women carry within themselves the capacity for great pain, the capacity for great joy, and the tenacity to glide seamlessly between both. Surprisingly, a woman's child bearing years are actually quite brief if you look at the numbers - most women live another 40 years after menopause - even though it rarely feels that way.

Truth be told, we have all been sold a narrative that has not only hindered us in our feminine journey but it has harmed many along the way. We have been misguided by the outdated patriarchal notion that we are no longer *useful* as women once we hit menopause. Nothing could be further from the reality of our gender. Women are naturally drawn to purpose. Whether we find that purpose in the care of others or in the many passions we pursue in life, women do not cease to contribute to society simply because their reproductive window has drawn to a close. On the contrary, women often find even more ways to express themselves in action once they are postmenopausal. The ability to shift focus, to be adaptive and fully present, these are qualities we women embrace when menopause has run its course.

So what really is life like after menopause? Do you simply return to your premenopausal self or is there a different version of you waiting to be realized? Is the journey of womanhood at an end?

Life after menopause is very much like arriving at the promised land. After years of wading through discomfort and ever-shifting changes, you have reached the land of surety in yourself. Though many women claim back a very big part of who they were before menopause, most share that they are decidedly different people after menopause - and that they wouldn't have it any other way. My friends, colleagues, and family members all share the same insight: I know myself more. I'm more confident as a woman and as a person. I just don't put up with nonsense the way I used to. In other words, they have reached the best part of womanhood and they feel - as do I - that this is simply the realization of our journey and we are nowhere close to its end.

WHEN DO YOU KNOW YOU'VE MADE IT?

Strictly speaking, being post-menopausal is defined as the period that commences after you have not had a menstrual cycle for 12 consecutive months. Many women start to experience the relief of being post-menopausal before this 12 month mark, and already share in the joys of the experience during the months in which menopause draws to a close.

To recap, there are three stages to menopause:

Perimenopause - the stage that leads up to menopause, often the stage confused with the term menopause, during which hormones decline and your menstrual cycle becomes erratic and irregular. Most side effects of menopause occur during this early stage already such as vaginal dryness, night sweats, or hot flashes.

Menopause - the stage at which your body has stopped producing the hormone levels that create your menstrual period for 12 months (the tipping point).

Postmenopause - the period after which you have not had a menstrual period for 12 months.

I like to think of postmenopause as the celebration era in which you explore an entirely new chapter in your life. My spiritual guide and confidant revealed to me that being a postmenopausal woman is the stage of your life that has been promised to you as a gift for all the work that you and your amazing body did in earlier years. It is the most feminine stage of your life - because being a fully empowered goddess-like force of nature is far more female than simply the ability to reproduce. We are more than just our reproductive organs. We are women - and that is the magic of what we become.

For others, menopause is merely another facet of life. In fact, a close friend of mine, Mimi, had the best thing to say about Menopause. She said: I didn't suffer from menopause. I went through it, but I didn't suffer. When I asked her how she coped so easily, she explained that it wasn't about things being easier for her than others, it's that "I just worked with it.".

On the other hand, my sweet aunty, Leona, had the absolute worst experience. Every symptom plagued her with maximum effect, she had profuse sweating even for years after her menses stopped. She had bouts of hot flashes so intense she would be whimpering and dizzy from the experience. After so many years of struggle, she is now bubbly and in control again. It took her a long time to figure out her body's needs and to address the hormonal balance she lacked. Now that she has, she feels like a new person.

So how do you know with absolute certainty that you have made it? Well, as we have discussed, the definitive requirement for being considered postmenopausal is not having a menstrual cycle or bleeding for at least a year. However, your healthcare provider can take a blood sample to check your hormone level and confirm that you have actually completed your journey through menopause. Other signs will be based on your symptoms, though these are not as accurate, there are still a few lingering symptoms that last well into postmenopause.

Let's explore what being postmenopausal looks like and the symptoms you should be expecting. First and foremost, we need to acknowledge that no human being exists solely in one state or another like a binary switch - we are not robots. We gradually evolve from one state to another and continue to do so over the years with varying levels of hormones, age, and even lifestyle events, all playing a part in our wellness and condition. This means two main things: one - no one person's menopause journey is going to be the exact same and two - your symptoms will evolve and shift as a part of the process, not as on/off indicators to say 'now you are experiencing menopause and now you are not'.

Symptoms you can expect during postmenopause include:

- Hot flashes
- Night sweats

- Depression
- Vaginal dryness
- Sexual discomfort
- Changes in sex drive
- Insomnia
- Hair loss
- Weight changes
- Urinary incontinence
- Dry skin

Remember, many of these symptoms are still carried over from perimenopause though they generally decline in intensity and for many stop altogether. Symptoms are based on your low reproductive hormone levels and should be addressed accordingly.

This also means that using your symptoms as an indicator of when you have hit the postmenopausal mark is inconclusive and unreliable - but it is useful to note the degree of severity these symptoms have, in order to know more about where you are in your menopause journey.

What are the risks associated with being postmenopause?

There are a number of risks associated with being postmenopausal that I find are all too often glossed over and simply not discussed. The problem is that there is so much information on hot sweats or mood swings but not enough on the very real risks connected to low estrogen levels. Some of the conditions you have an increased risk of due to menopause include: cardiovascular disease, osteoporosis, vaginal atrophy, and mental health issues.

So what can you do? Apart from the advice that I've given under each condition, the general consensus with regards to risk factors caused by menopause is that you should continue living your life in the best manner possible and ensure that you are taking care of your wellness and health. Healthy diet, exercise, supplements (when appropriate), no smoking, and seeking help when and where you need it - that is what you should be doing to empower yourself during your postmenopausal journey.

DOES LIFE GO BACK TO NORMAL AFTER MENOPAUSE?

The only truthful answer I can give to this question is perhaps frustratingly dappled. Will life ever go back to normal? Yes and no.

No, you will probably never feel the same way you did before menopause and there is a certain sadness to that. You might even mourn the loss of who you once were pre-menopause - the self that you had cultivated through most of your adult life (so far). Menopause can also affect your perception of normal - During perimenopause, you may frequently experience hot flashes, mood swings, and other symptoms, creating a sense of chaos and imbalance. Plus, there is the reality that you will never be able to undo what is being done, However, there is beauty and grace in this transition. Embracing the journey of menopause and the process of aging can lead to a more fulfilling experience.

On the opposite side of the coin, I can tell you that, YES! You will feel normal again. Note that I did not say 'the same as before'; instead, you will find a new normal that makes sense for you. The caveat here, of course, is that it will take quite a few years until you reach a state of being postmenopausal and that while you are in the thick of it, it may feel as if normal will never exist again. Fear not. Things will start to make sense again as menopause draws to a close, and then you have the most exciting time ahead to look forward to life as a postmenopausal woman.

You will certainly feel *different* after menopause - and that is a GOOD THING. Your hormones will be different, you will have gained a few years of age and experience, and you will have transformed yourself and your relationships (hopefully all in a positive way).

The best news? If you look after yourself properly during menopause, you may even feel better than you did before menopause. So not only will you feel normal again, but you will feel surprised about the positive effect it has had on your life. Now, doesn't that sound like something to look forward to?

LET'S GET TO THE GOOD PART!

We have explored quite extensively all the side effects and symptoms that you can expect not only as part and parcel of menopause but also what you should anticipate during your postmenopausal journey. What about the promise of it all being worth it? Let's get to the good part: here are the best parts and benefits to look forward to once you have made it to the bonus round: postmenopause.

You could be having the best sex of your life. Okay, I know I started with a really good one, but after everything you go through during menopause, I think we deserve a little bit of sexual and sensual fun, and so does Mother Nature. In fact, studies have shown that about 67% of women over the age of 65 are having orgasms "most of the time" or "always" during sex. Sounds good? It gets better: the eldest women in the study were found not only to be the most sexually satisfied overall but they were experiencing orgasm satisfaction rates similar to the youngest participants in the study.

You will feel more confident. I'm not going to say this has anything to do with the last point I made… but it doesn't hurt. On top of that, women who have gone through menopause often reach a sense of satisfaction, pride, and happiness with their physical appearance unperturbed by the effects of hormones and age. In fact, surveys show that women over 55 are the most confident wearing beachwear. This is a testament to the knowledge and experience of older women, who have embraced the fullness of their feminine energy after reaching postmenopause.

You might experience fewer colds. This observation might seem unexpected, but it's linked to the aging process that coincides with menopause. Over the years, your immune system has encountered numerous viruses, making it stronger and more resilient. As you move past menopause and your body adjusts to hormonal changes, it can more effectively focus on maintaining your health without the added strain of fluctuating hormones.

You can enjoy more freedom. Retirement often coincides with menopause (sometimes these are linked, as we explored in earlier chapters, and other times they are not), which allows you more free time - plain and simple. Once menopause has run its course, you can enjoy time spent with friends, travel, take up new hobbies, and basically enjoy yourself as fully as possible, unencumbered by the effects of menopause.

You will sleep better. Night sweats can wreak havoc on anyone's sleep patterns, and hormone fluctuations don't exactly create a picture of perfect rest either. Sleep improves when you reach post-menopause, as does the quality of your rest.

Your memory will improve. This may come in handy as you reach your golden years - a stronger memory unhindered by the effects of menopause. Forgetfulness, fogginess, and overall fugue state all seem to clear up when menopause comes to a close. While many women suffer a decline in memory during menopause, it does appear to be temporary for most, and your memory could return to pre-menopausal levels during postmenopause.

So, there really is light at the end of the tunnel. The rainbow after the hormone storm, if you will. Remember, I'm saying this based on numerous accounts from women who have experienced menopause; one clear message emerges: Embracing your authentic self and living true to who you are becomes even more powerful once you've navigated through the menopause journey.

So what now?

What happens once you have gone through all of the harrowing symptoms and experiences that menopause has to offer and come out on the other side ready for the good, better, and best part of the journey? Well, for some women, it provides them a renewed energy for pursuing the passions they may have felt too overwhelming during the perimenopause stage. For others, it is time for a dramatic life change in which they may choose to sell their house, pack up, and travel the world in a camper van or even take on a new vocation such as coaching or writing. Some women take post-menopause as a time to nurture and give back - to their families and greater communities. Some women simply just enjoy finally having some peace and quiet.

The key question isn't what you're supposed to do after reaching postmenopause. Rather, it's: what do you want to do now?

This is YOUR time. Your body, mind, and spirit have experienced a significant transformation. As with every major shift in life, this period should be celebrated. From maidenhood, marked by first kisses, high school crushes, and your time driving, to motherhood with its baby showers, first words, and sleepless nights preparing for birthdays, you've journeyed to your current stage of womanhood. Now, it's up to you to define what this phase means and how you want to celebrate this remarkable period of your life. So, what's next? It's time to go out and fully live this experience.

Case Study: The Inspirational Story of Indiana

My friend Indiana was a dancer all her life and maintained excellent health and nutritional habits. She also grew up in a community where most of the people around her believed in taking pills prescribed by doctors or going for operations wherever something wasn't right with their bodies. When she hit perimenopause, she started experiencing many of the symptoms we have already discussed, so she went to their family doctor, who placed her on hormone replacement therapy. She was told that would fix everything, and she would get back to feeling herself again. She took the medication home and decided to take it; after all, the doctors know best. She took it for a week, but her body did not respond well. Suddenly, on top of the menopause symptoms she had, she started getting regular headaches, breast pain, or tenderness, feeling nauseated all the time.

After 2 weeks on the medication, she decided to start looking for alternatives; she realized that the pills were not going to 'solve her problem.' She read a couple of books and spoke to a friend who was an expert in holistic healing. She started incorporating regular acupuncture, moderate exercise in the form of daily walks, and more and more mindfulness practices like breathing, meditation, and yoga into her life. She also set aside time daily to take care of her emotional world, journaling and allowing herself time to acknowledge and process her feelings and emotions. On top of this, she made changes to her diet, incorporating more fruits and vegetables and avoiding caffeine, sugar, and alcohol altogether.

After a month or so, she started feeling better, her vitality returned, and today, she is the picture of health and serenity; her skin is always glowing, and she radiates peace and joy. Her figure would make most 25-year-olds a little jealous, and she enjoys a happy sex life with her husband.

Whenever I think of Indiana, I know that it is entirely possible to manage your body through this change without putting yourself at risk by taking artificial hormones and other medication to 'fix the problem.' I hope that sharing this story will also help you through the challenging stages of menopause and assist you in formulating a menopause mastery plan that works for YOU!

Thank you so much for reaching this point in the book. If it's been a positive journey for you, I'd be grateful if you could share your experience by leaving a review on Amazon.

Taking 60 seconds of your time to share your thoughts can significantly impact someone else's journey, offering them the support and strategies they need to thrive this universal transition.

Thank you so much for considering to pay it forward with your review.

Kindly scan the QR code below or use the link to leave a review.

https://www.amazon.com/review/create-review?&asin=B0CX1G1WXF

CONCLUSION

If you have come to this point in this book, congratulations! You have already done more for yourself than what most women do when it comes to menopause mastery and you are now equipped with a thorough body of information that you can use to navigate this journey.

In this book, we have looked at everything menopause-related, and we did so from a fresh, modern perspective, with the sole purpose of empowering you.

In chapter 1, I demystified menopause for you, showing you how it is a natural metamorphosis, and I simplified the scientific aspects of menopause while also sharing with you why menopause is important, including its history, biology, and the evolutionary advantage of menopause

In the next chapter, we looked at the science of menopause, an in-depth exploration of both common and less-discussed symptoms of menopause, and I gave you some of my best insights, advice, and solutions to help you navigate this transformative life stage.

Chapter 3 dealt with the profound emotional and psychological components of menopause, and in this part of the book, we delved deep into understanding and managing the emotional ups and downs of menopause, and I equipped you with actionable strategies for mental wellness.

Chapter 4 is all about navigating the relationship challenges that come with menopause, while Chapter 5 opened up a world of holistic approaches for managing menopause, giving you options for a more comprehensive, personalized, and natural way to address the physical, emotional, and mental changes of menopause.

In Chapter 6, we took a deep dive into how you have to use the food you eat every day to help you feel better. I introduced the empowering idea of using food as medicine, an excellent idea for the whole family, not just the menopausal woman, and finally, in chapter 7, I revealed to you how the need for menopause can become your own personal promised land!

We have certainly covered a lot of ground together, and I want to leave you now with a reminder that, while menopause is universal, every person experiences it differently and it is never too late to take charge of your body and your health. Even small changes, like taking up some light exercise or spending 10 minutes every morning just checking in with yourself, can start to move the needle towards a healthier, more fulfilling menopause journey. You don't have to get it right the first time, remember, perfect is the enemy of done. Just get started today and you will thank yourself in the future.

One of the most powerful things I have learned through my own journey is that, like with many things in life, the beauty is in the eye of the beholder and the way you frame this journey in your mind, will directly impact how you experience it.

By now, we have seen enough evidence, with more and more coming out every week, to understand that our mental state affects our physical bodies. When you really believe this, your mind becomes your best friend in this journey.

Just the other day a friend was talking about hot flashes, and I told her that I actually quite enjoy them. I had started tuning in to the sensations of the hot flashes as they came on, and in my mind, I started looking forward to the tingling, warm sensation. My friend couldn't believe what she was hearing, but since that day, my hot flashes have become much easier to manage, and I have really started enjoying it and looking at it with a sense of curiosity and wonder instead of judgment and fear.

I encourage you to view this journey as an adventure, and an opportunity to get to know yourself better. A chance to experiment with new experiences, new foods, and new practices, to find out what works for you.

May you have a wonderful journey ahead, and may you find fulfillment and joy in the unfolding of this magical chapter of your life.

Yours in Menopause Mastery,

Maya Bloom

NOTES

1. THE MENOPAUSE METAMORPHOSIS - WHAT REALLY HAPPENS?

1. https://www.sciencedirect.com/science/article/pii/S0015028216578492
2. https://www.ncbi.nlm.nih.gov/pmc/articles/PMC5888979/#:~:text=Life style%20factors%20such%20as%20smoking,ovarian%20germ%20cells%20(16).
3. https://www.uclahealth.org/news/menopause-sleepless-nights-may-make-women-age-faster

2. SYMPTOM SPECTRUM - FROM MILD TO WILD

1. https://www.statista.com/statistics/1242168/womens-knowledge-awareness-perimenopause-menopause-worldwide/
2. https://www.ncbi.nlm.nih.gov/pmc/articles/PMC3322543/

3. NAVIGATE THE EMOTIONAL ROLLERCOASTER

1. https://www.health.harvard.edu/healthbeat/giving-thanks-can-make-you-happier#:~:text=In%20positive%20psychology%20research%2C%20gratitude,adversity%2C%20and%20build%20strong%20relationships
2. https://pubmed.ncbi.nlm.nih.gov/35486946/

4. SAILING SMOOTH - RELATIONSHIPS & MENOPAUSE

1. https://www.gov.uk/government/publications/menopause-transition-effects-on-womens-economic-participation

5. NATURE'S NURTURING - HOLISTIC HEALING

1. https://www.ncbi.nlm.nih.gov/pmc/articles/PMC3555027/
2. https://www.tandfonline.com/doi/abs/10.1080/13697137.2018.1551344?journalCode=icmt20
3. https://www.ncbi.nlm.nih.gov/pmc/articles/PMC3679190/
4. https://www.contemporaryobgyn.net/view/therapeutic-touch-and-music-improve-sleep-during-menopause
5. https://www.balancehormoneoklahoma.com/blog/the-history-of-menopause
6. https://www.frontiersin.org/articles/10.3389/fmed.2022.1043390/full

BIBLIOGRAPHY

The emotional roller coaster of menopause. (2002, October 6). WebMD. https://www.webmd.com/menopause/emotional-roller-coaster

Menopause & Motherhood: Raising children while menopausal. (n.d.). A.Vogel Talks Menopause. https://www.avogel.co.uk/health/menopause/videos/menopause-motherhood-raising-children-while-menopausal/

balance menopause. (2023, March 21). *Why children are the forgotten victims of menopause - balance menopause.* Balance Menopause. https://www.balance-menopause.com/menopause-library/why-children-are-the-forgotten-victims-of-menopause/#:~:text=The%20most%20common%20menopausal%20symptoms,when%20irritable%20or%20in%20pain.

Southside Medical Center. (n.d.). *10 Menopause Care Tips: How to Take Care of Yourself During Menopause.* Retrieved January 29, 2024, from https://southsidemedical.net/how-do-i-take-care-of-myself-during-menopause-10-menopause-care-tips/

CIPD | The menopause at work: guidance for line managers. (n.d.). CIPD. https://www.cipd.org/uk/knowledge/guides/menopause-people-manager-guidance/

Girvin, J. (2023, December 19). *Everything I needed to know about the menopause. . . No One Told Me - Evidently Cochrane.* Evidently Cochrane. https://www.evidentlycochrane.net/everything-needed-know-menopause-no-one-told/

LinkedIn Login, Sign in | LinkedIn. (n.d.). LinkedIn. https://www.linkedin.com/pulse/silent-struggle-unveiling-effects-menopause-tracy-kimberg-/

Menopause symptoms. (n.d.). WebMD. https://www.webmd.com/menopause/ss/slideshow-10-ways-to-deal-with-menopause-symptoms

Dineanddiet. (2023, June 29). Self-Care for Relationships: How to Build Healthy Relationships with Yourself and Others. *Medium.* https://medium.com/@dineanddiet/self-care-for-relationships-how-to-build-healthy-relationships-with-yourself-and-others-2f7ca0d3d629

The Health Benefits of Social Support during the Menopausal Transition. (n.d.). https://www.menopausenaturalsolutions.com/blog/social-support

Naworska, B., & Brzęk, A. (2020). The Relationship between Health Status and Social Activity of Perimenopausal and Postmenopausal Women (Health Status and Social Relationships in Menopause). *International Journal of Environmental Research and Public Health,* 17(22), 8388. https://doi.org/10.3390/ijerph17228388

Menopause and mental health: finding yourself in isolation. (n.d.). https://www.gennev.

com/education/social-isolation-menopause-mental-health#:~:text=It's%20im portant%20to%20take%20the,and%20call%20up%20a%20friend.
Mariette. (2023, August 30). *Menopause in the Workplace - Women's Health Concern*. Women's Health Concern. https://www.womens-health-concern.org/help-and-advice/menopause-in-the-workplace/#:~:text=The%20most%20com monly%20reported%20difficulties,intention%20to%20leave%20the%20work force.
Misiaszek, A. B. a. T. (2023, December 21). Viewpoint: Understanding the impact of menopause in the workplace. *SHRM*. https://www.shrm.org/resourcesand tools/hr-topics/behavioral-competencies/global-and-cultural-effectiveness/ pages/viewpoint-understanding-the-impact-of-menopause-in-the-workplace.aspx
CIPD | Menopause in the workplace. (n.d.). CIPD. https://www.cipd.org/en/knowl edge/reports/menopause-workplace-experiences/
Government Equalities Office. (2017, July 20). *Menopause transition: effects on women's economic participation*. GOV.UK. https://www.gov.uk/government/ publications/menopause-transition-effects-on-womens-economic-participation
Garlick, D. (n.d.). *Menopause and work: why it's so important – Menopause in the Workplace | Henpicked*. https://menopauseintheworkplace.co.uk/articles/ menopause-and-work-its-important/
The National Council on Aging. (n.d.). https://www.ncoa.org/article/how-does-menopause-affect-women-at-work
Business Bliss FZE. (2023, November 6). *Psych-social changes in middle adulthood*. https://www.ukessays.com/essays/psychology/psychsocial-changes-in-middle.php
Hardy, C., Thorne, E., Griffiths, A., & Hunter, M. (2018). Work outcomes in midlife women: the impact of menopause, work stress and working environment. *Women's Midlife Health*, 4(1). https://doi.org/10.1186/s40695-018-0036-z
Letts, R. (2022, July 19). *Mood changes during menopause – does what you eat make a difference?* Health & Her. https://healthandher.com/expert-advice/low-mood/ mood-changes-during-menopausedoes-what-you-eat-make-a-difference/#:~: text=Researchers%20suspect%20that%20GABA%20may,brown%20rice% 20and%20nutritional%20yeast.
British Journal of Nursing - Nutrition during the menopause: clinical considerations. (n.d.). British Journal of Nursing. https://www.britishjournalofnursing.com/content/ comment/nutrition-during-the-menopause-clinical-considerations/#:~:text= Women%20can%20lose%20up%20to,are%20all%20made%20of%20protein.
DeAngelis, T. (n.d.). *Menopause can be rough. Psychology is here to help*.

https://www.apa.org. https://www.apa.org/monitor/2023/09/easing-transition-into-menopause

Kalra, B., Agarwal, S., & Magon, S. (2012). Holistic care of menopause: Understanding the framework. *Journal of Mid-life Health, 3*(2), 66. https://doi.org/10.4103/0976-7800.104453

Wattar, B. H. A., & Talaulikar, V. (2023). Non-oestrogen-based and complementary therapies for menopause. *Best Practice & Research Clinical Endocrinology & Metabolism*, 101819. https://doi.org/10.1016/j.beem.2023.101819

Lac, E. H. (2023, April 13). *Holistic Guide to Managing Stress & Finding balance.* Awakened Path Counseling. https://www.awakenedpathcounseling.com/holistic-guide-to-managing-stress/#:~:text=Holistic%20stress%20management%20is%20essential,to%20mental%20and%20physical%20health.

NESTA Personal Trainer Certification, Nutrition Courses, Fitness Education. (2022, October 28). *Major factors to consider in a holistic lifestyle.* Personal Trainer Certification, Nutrition Courses, Fitness Education. https://www.nestacertified.com/major-factors-to-consider-in-a-holistic-lifestyle/

Rabago, P. (2022, April 11). *16 Holistic Lifestyle tips: How to create one for yourself.* First Day Life Inc. https://firstday.com/blogs/news/16-holistic-lifestyle-tips-how-to-create-one-for-yourself#:~:text=One%20of%20the%20best%20ways,exercising%2C%20and%20getting%20enough%20sleep.

What is holistic health? Overview and career outcomes. (2022, May 20). https://www.stkate.edu/healthcare-degrees/what-is-holistic-health#:~:text=Holistic%20health%20is%20an%20approach,communities%2C%20and%20even%20the%20environment.

Waltz, N. (2022, September 12). *The history of menopause.* Tabu Group. https://www.heytabu.com/blogs/mentionables/the-history-of-menopause

Menopause treatments that can relieve your symptoms: ageless restoration: alternative medicine. (n.d.). https://www.balancehormoneoklahoma.com/blog/menopause-treatments-that-can-relieve-your-symptoms

Seo, R. D. (n.d.). *» Herbal remedies traditionally used for treating menopause.* https://www.menopausecentre.com.au/information-centre/articles/herbal-remedies-for-treating-menopause/

Herbal Remedies for Menopause, Menopause information & articles | The North American Menopause Society, NAMS. (n.d.). https://www.menopause.org/for-women/menopauseflashes/menopause-symptoms-and-treatments/natural-remedies-for-hot-flashes

Mundy, L. (2022, October 28). The secret power of menopause. *The Atlantic.* https://www.theatlantic.com/magazine/archive/2019/10/the-secret-power-of-menopause/596662/

Women First. (2022, October). *The Next Chapter.* Retrieved January 29, 2024, from https://www.womenfirst.com/wp-content/uploads/2022/10/The_Next_Chapter_Proof-English.pdf

Whn. (2023, February 28). *Menopause in different cultures.* Women's Health Network. https://www.womenshealthnetwork.com/menopause-and-perimenopause/menopause-in-different-cultures/

Iqbal, J., & Zaidi, M. (2009). Understanding Estrogen Action during Menopause. *Endocrinology, 150*(8), 3443–3445. https://doi.org/10.1210/en.2009-0449

Estrogen's effects on the female body. (2022, November 1). Johns Hopkins Medicine. https://www.hopkinsmedicine.org/health/conditions-and-diseases/estrogens-effects-on-the-female-body

Professional, C. C. M. (n.d.). *Low estrogen.* Cleveland Clinic. https://my.clevelandclinic.org/health/diseases/22354-low-estrogen

Professional, C. C. M. (n.d.-b). *Progesterone.* Cleveland Clinic. https://my.clevelandclinic.org/health/body/24562-progesterone

Early or premature menopause | Office on Women's Health. (n.d.). https://www.womenshealth.gov/menopause/early-or-premature-menopause

Professional, C. C. M. (n.d.-b). *Postmenopause.* Cleveland Clinic. https://my.clevelandclinic.org/health/diseases/21837-postmenopause

Postmenopause. (2024, January 5). University of Utah Health | University of Utah Health. https://healthcare.utah.edu/womens-health/gynecology/menopause/postmenopause

Scaccia, A. (2023, June 30). *How long do symptoms of menopause last?* Healthline. https://www.healthline.com/health/menopause/how-long-does-menopause-last#symptoms

Davis, S. R., & Wåhlin-Jacobsen, S. (2015). Testosterone in women—the clinical significance. *The Lancet Diabetes & Endocrinology, 3*(12), 980–992. https://doi.org/10.1016/s2213-8587(15)00284-3

Professional, C. C. M. (n.d.-b). *Low testosterone in women.* Cleveland Clinic. https://my.clevelandclinic.org/health/diseases/24897-low-testosterone-in-women

Pietrangelo, A. (2017, May 4). *Can you get pregnant after menopause?* Healthline. https://www.healthline.com/health/menopause/menopause-pregnancy

Cramer, D. W., Xu, H., & Harlow, B. L. (1995). Family history as a predictor of early menopause. *Fertility and Sterility, 64*(4), 740–745. https://doi.org/10.1016/s0015-0282(16)57849-2

Whitcomb, B. W., Purdue-Smithe, A., Szegda, K., Boutot, M. E., Hankinson, S. E., Manson, J. E., Rosner, B., Willett, W. C., Eliassen, A. H., & Bertone-Johnson, E. R. (2017). Cigarette smoking and risk of early natural menopause. *American Journal of Epidemiology, 187*(4), 696–704. https://doi.org/10.1093/aje/kwx292

Hysterectomy increases risk for earlier menopause among younger women, study finds. (2011, November 11). ScienceDaily. https://www.sciencedaily.com/releases/2011/11/111114112311.htm

Menopause, sleepless nights may make women age faster. (n.d.). UCLA Health. https://www.uclahealth.org/news/menopause-sleepless-nights-may-make-women-age-faster

Hot flashes - Symptoms & causes - Mayo Clinic. (2023, December 12). Mayo Clinic. https://www.mayoclinic.org/diseases-conditions/hot-flashes/symptoms-causes/syc-20352790

The History of Menopause: Ageless Restoration: Alternative Medicine. (n.d.). https://www.balancehormoneoklahoma.com/blog/the-history-of-menopause

How does menopause affect my sleep? (2021, August 8). Johns Hopkins Medicine. https://www.hopkinsmedicine.org/health/wellness-and-prevention/how-does-menopause-affect-my-sleep

How sex changes after Menopause. (2023, October 30). Johns Hopkins Medicine. https://www.hopkinsmedicine.org/health/wellness-and-prevention/how-sex-changes-after-menopause#:~:text=Your%20estrogen%20takes%20a%20nosedive,for%20you%20to%20become%20aroused.

Harvard Health. (2021, August 17). *Don't ignore vaginal dryness and pain.* https://www.health.harvard.edu/womens-health/dont-ignore-vaginal-dryness-and-pain

Many women have cognition issues during menopause. (n.d.). UCLA Health. https://www.uclahealth.org/news/many-women-have-cognition-issues-during-menopause#:~:text=Although%20the%20reasons%20for%20menopause,believed%20to%20play%20a%20role.

Society, E. (2022, January 24). *Menopause and bone loss.* Endocrine Society. https://www.endocrine.org/patient-engagement/endocrine-library/menopause-and-bone-loss#:~:t

Society, E. (2022b, January 24). *Menopause and bone loss.* Endocrine Society. https://www.endocrine.org/patient-engagement/endocrine-library/menopause-and-bone-loss#:~:text=As%20hormones%20change%20to%20accommodate,significantly%20speeds%20up%20bone%20loss.

Menopause basics | Office on Women's Health. (n.d.). https://www.womenshealth.gov/menopause/menopause-basics#:~:text=Menopause%20is%20when%20your%20period%20stops%20permanently.&text=It%20is%20sometimes%20called%20%22the,the%20United%20States%20is%2052.

Irregular periods and menopause. (n.d.). https://www.avogel.co.uk/health/menopause/symptoms/irregular-periods/

Iqbal, J., & Zaidi, M. (2009b). Understanding Estrogen Action during Menopause. *Endocrinology, 150*(8), 3443–3445. https://doi.org/10.1210/en.2009-0449

Heitkemper, M., & Chang, L. (2009). Do fluctuations in ovarian hormones affect gastrointestinal symptoms in women with irritable bowel syndrome? *Gender Medicine, 6,* 152–167. https://doi.org/10.1016/j.genm.2009.03.004

Digestive problems and menopause. (n.d.). https://www.avogel.co.uk/health/

menopause/symptoms/digestive-problems/

Magliano, M. (2010). Menopausal arthralgia: Fact or fiction. *Maturitas, 67*(1), 29–33. https://doi.org/10.1016/j.maturitas.2010.04.009

Sex hormones and headache. (2000). PubMed. https://pubmed.ncbi.nlm.nih.gov/11139745/

5 eye problems to look out for during menopause. (n.d.). A.Vogel Talks Menopause. https://www.avogel.co.uk/health/menopause/videos/5-eye-problems-to-look-out-for-during-menopause/

Menopause & Urinary Symptoms | CU Urogynecology | Colorado. (2020, June 18). University of Colorado Urogynecology. https://urogyn.coloradowomenshealth.com/conditions/bladder/menopause-urinary-symptoms.html#:~:text=Causes%20of%20menopausal%20urinary%20symptoms&text=The%20lack%20of%20estrogen%20weakens,ability%20to%20control%20urinary%20functions.

Alexander, H. (2020, June 5). What are macronutrients? *MD Anderson Cancer Center.* https://www.mdanderson.org/publications/focused-on-health/what-are-macronutrients-.h15-1593780.html#:~:text=Carbohydrates%2C%20fat%20and%20protein%20are,Anderson%20Wellness%20Dietitian%20Lindsey%20Wohlford.

Nemours KidsHealth. (2021, January). *Vitamins and Minerals.* Retrieved January 29, 2024, from https://kidshealth.org/en/teens/vitamins-minerals.html

How to manage inflammation during menopause. (n.d.). https://www.feistymenopause.com/blog/Manage-Inflammation-During-Menopause

Sugar and menopause: the two don't mix. (n.d.). https://www.gennev.com/education/sugar-and-menopause

DeMaio, K. B. (2023, December 13). Exactly what happens to your hair during menopause. *Oprah Daily.* https://www.oprahdaily.com/beauty/hair/a40517158/menopause-hair-loss-thinning-treatment/

Rd, R. a. M. (2020, January 17). *What are functional foods? All you need to know.* Healthline. https://www.healthline.com/nutrition/functional-foods#examples

Sissons, C. (2023, December 22). *Typical testosterone levels in males and females.* https://www.medicalnewstoday.com/articles/323085

Catya_Shok. (2017, March 29). *Cute summer butterfly.* iStock. https://www.istockphoto.com/vector/summer-butterfly-watercolor-illustration-gm659645624-120420635

Made in the USA
Monee, IL
11 July 2024